The Preceptor's Handbook for Supervising Physician Assistants

Randy Danielsen, PhD, PA-C
Emeritus Professor
A.T. Still University
Senior Vice-President
National Commission on Certification of
Physician Assistants Foundation

Ruth Ballweg, MPA, PA-C
Associate Professor and Division Chief
University of Washington MEDEX Program
Chair, Board of Trustees
Group Health Cooperative

Linda Vorvick, MD
Medical Director and Lecturer
University of Washington MEDEX Program

Donald Sefcik, DO, MBA
Senior Associate Dean
Michigan State University College of Osteopathic Medicine

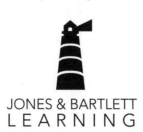

JONES & BARTLETT
L E A R N I N G

World Headquarters

Jones & Bartlett Learning
40 Tall Pine Drive
Sudbury, MA 01776
978-443-5000
info@jblearning.com
www.jblearning.com

Jones & Bartlett Learning
Canada
6339 Ormindale Way
Mississauga, Ontario L5V 1J2
Canada

Jones & Bartlett Learning
International
Barb House, Barb Mews
London W6 7PA
United Kingdom

Jones & Bartlett Learning books and products are available through most bookstores
and online booksellers. To contact Jones & Bartlett Learning directly, call 800-832-0034,
fax 978-443-8000, or visit our website, www.jblearning.com.

The authors, editor, and publisher have made every effort to provide accurate information. However, they are not responsible for errors, omissions, or for any outcomes related to the use of the contents of this book and take no responsibility for the use of the products and procedures described. Treatments and side effects described in this book may not be applicable to all people; likewise, some people may require a dose or experience a side effect that is not described herein. Drugs and medical devices are discussed that may have limited availability controlled by the Food and Drug Administration (FDA) for use only in a research study or clinical trial. Research, clinical practice, and government regulations often change the accepted standard in this field. When consideration is being given to use of any drug in the clinical setting, the health care provider or reader is responsible for determining FDA status of the drug, reading the package insert, and reviewing prescribing information for the most up-to-date recommendations on dose, precautions, and contraindications, and determining the appropriate usage for the product. This is especially important in the case of drugs that are new or seldom used.

Production Credits

Publisher: David D. Cella
Acquisitions Editor: Katey Birtcher
Associate Editor: Maro Gartside
Editorial Assistant: Teresa Reilly
Senior Production Editor: Renée Sekerak
Production Assistant: Sean Coombs
Marketing Manager: Grace Richards

Manufacturing and Inventory Control
    Supervisor: Amy Bacus
Cover Design: Scott Moden
Cover Image: © Yuri Arcurs/ShutterStock, Inc.
Composition: Cenveo Publisher Services
Printing and Binding: Malloy, Inc.
Cover Printing: Malloy, Inc.

Library of Congress Cataloging-in-Publication Data

The preceptor's handbook for supervising physician assistants / Randy
Danielsen ... [et al.].
    p. ; cm.
 Includes bibliographical references and index.
 ISBN 978-0-7637-7361-8 (pbk.)
 1. Physicians' assistants. 2. Nursing—Study and teaching
(Preceptorship). 3. Supervision. I. Danielsen, Randy.
 [DNLM: 1. Physician Assistants—education. 2.
Preceptorship—organization & administration. W 20]
 R697.P45P74 2012
 610.73'72069—dc22

                                                      2011001887
6048

Printed in the United States of America
15 14 13 12   10 9 8 7 6 5 4 3 2

This book is dedicated to all physicians who support physician assistants by being advocates, policy makers, educators, supervising physicians, and preceptors for students. We appreciate your time, guidance, and support.

This book is also dedicated to physician assistants and nurse practitioners who are clinical preceptors and role models. Your efforts have made the difference.

Contents

Foreword

The physician assistant (PA) concept responds to many needs. This timely and much needed book emphasizes the fact that this concept is an innovation originated by physicians based on a continuing and expanding relationship between the PA and a specific physician supervisor. Physicians who understand this relationship also understand and accept the obligations and responsibilities implicit in this role as well as the advantages to themselves, the PA, and their mutual patients, which flow from its proper implementation. It is my observation that this role is accepted and valued by most physicians and PAs, but it is not one to be automatically assumed, nor can it be viewed as fully understood by all. Each relationship is unique, and, like a healthy marriage, requires constant attention and effort from all involved. The advantages of this relationship include the flexibility to expand roles, to innovate, and to solve problems in unique ways, without requiring changes in statutes or licenses. This will be even more apparent as we face the expanded eligibility of all our citizens under the recently enacted Health Reform Act of 2010.

—**E. Harvey Estes, MD**
Professor Emeritus
Community and Family Medicine
Duke University Medical Center
Durham, NC

Physician supervision has been key to the physician assistant (PA) concept from its beginning. It is the linkage underlying the profession's conception, its growing positive image, its acceptance by doctors, and the confidence patients and their families have had in the movement since it began more than four decades ago. Supervision has also been extremely important to the continued growth of the profession because it drives continuous improvement in the care possible with the collaborative team relationship fostered in the physician–PA setting. Knowing that a PA and physician are in a mutually supportive relationship provides patients with the comforting knowledge that the PA provides—or develops a direct pathway for—the best possible care in their environment. Knowledge of the supervisory relationship provides patients, doctors, and administrators with the knowledge and confidence that the health care being provided by physician assistants is helping our nation move forward in strengthening health care for all of our people.

—**Richard A. Smith, MD, MPH**
Developer of the MEDEX Concept
Founder, MEDEX Northwest
University of Washington and MEDEX International
University of Hawaii

Preface

The physician assistant concept was created "by physicians ... for physicians" to quote Dr. Richard Smith, one of the founders of the profession. Forty years later, the physician assistant role has grown and expanded—often due to the strong support of physician groups and individual physicians.

Despite that 40-year history, a lack of clarity sometimes remains in the minds of physicians, administrators, and other colleagues about how (and why) physicians and physician assistants work together. Other groups—such as nurse practitioners—have built their professional culture based on defining their own autonomy. Physician assistants, in contrast, see their relationship with physicians as the defining feature of the profession. As this book describes, physicians have felt comfortable with this type of supervisory relationship because it is consistent with the culture of medical education.

While the physician–physician assistant supervisory relationship is based on legal requirements, successful physician-PA teams work together based on relationships built over time. The recent physician-PA Teams Project developed by the National Commission on Certification of Physician Assistants Foundation (NCCPAF) identifies five features of effective physician-PA teams:

- Mutual trust and respect
- Shared priorities
- Frequent and effective communication

- Physician accessibility and approachability
- Consistency of delivery of patient care

In addition, the principles of team building (such as "delegate to strengths ... teach to weaknesses") also apply to the physician–PA relationship. Overall the physician–PA relationship is viewed as "dynamic," growing over time to benefit both individuals.

This guidebook is intended to assist all physicians—and healthcare systems—involved with PA utilization, supervision, and training. The first sections of the book provide information on the background of the profession and include information for the physician **preceptors** working with physician assistant students. The later sections of the book continue to discuss supervisory topics but also deal with issues more relevant for **supervisors** of physician assistants.

For the purpose of this publication, the term "preceptor" refers to the physician, or in some instances a nurse practitioner or graduate physician assistant, assigned to supervise physician assistant students during the clinical phase of their PA education. The term "supervising physician" refers to the physician who works with PAs in employment settings. In some cases that "supervising physician" may be the employer—although in large healthcare systems, the supervisor may also be the employee of the delivery system.

Acknowledging everyone's busy schedules in today's healthcare environment, the chapters in this book are purposely short and specific. The intent is that the reader be able to select a relevant topic and quickly gain an understanding of the issues.

In some chapters, case studies provide examples of possible supervisory situations.

Contributing Authors

James D. Cannon, MS, MBA, DHA, PA-C
Commander
U.S. Coast Guard
Consultant and Senior Physician Assistant
Contingency Medical Planning Health, Safety, and Work-Life
    Service Center
Norfolk, VA

James F. Cawley, MPH, PA-C
Professor and Vice-Chair
Department of Prevention and Community Health
School of Public Health and Health Services
The George Washington University
Washington, DC

Michael E. Goodwin, PA
Assistant Professor and Chair
Department of Physician Assistant Studies
Arizona School of Health Sciences
A.T. Still University
Mesa, AZ

Austin D. Potenza, JD
Attorney, Co-Founder
Collins, May, Potenza, Baran & Gillespie, PC
Phoenix, AZ

David Wayne, PhD
Coordinator
Academic Affairs
A.T. Still University
Mesa, AZ

An Introduction to the Profession

Chapter 1

Changing Healthcare Delivery Systems

THE US HEALTH SYSTEM

In most developed countries of the world, the government takes the lead role in the delivery of health care services. In the United States, the private sector plays a major role in the health system. Much of this is explained by the American traditions of self-reliance and avoidance of government regulation. Americans have steadfastly resisted attempts to establish the federal government as the controlling power of the healthcare system. This reliance on the private sector for the delivery of healthcare services has led to a patchwork of private and public systems of insurance coverage and services. Major healthcare services not adequately provided in the private sector include environmental protection, public health, support for biomedical research and training, and care for vulnerable populations; the US government has been most concerned and involved in these areas. Many of the characteristics of the US healthcare system are related to beliefs and values held dear by Americans—freedom, individualism, and capitalism.

Another feature of the US system is the centrality of the medical model, which emphasizes diagnosis and treatment of acute disease. This feature is the predominant mode of US healthcare services. Thus, prevention and health promotion tend to reflect individual behaviors rather than system-wide approaches. Reform of the US healthcare system has traditionally focused on the areas of cost, access, and quality. In the past decade significant changes have emerged in the tradition-bound and formerly physician-dominated healthcare system in this country. The next decade will do no less. This chapter presents a broad overview of the complex structures, processes, and relationships within the American healthcare system. It will also review how clinicians, particularly physician assistants (PAs), fit into the current and, perhaps, the future healthcare system in America.

MEASURES OF HEALTH CARE

Most would agree that the US healthcare system should provide affordable, high-quality healthcare services to everyone. For well over a half-century, and perhaps longer, cost, quality, and access have been the three key words measuring success. Healthcare now represents 17% of the gross national product (GNP), and it is estimated that more than 47 million Americans are either uninsured or underinsured. A debate continues regarding whether society (the government) has an obligation to ensure that all Americans have a right to health care and, if so, an obligation to make health care available to all. If the answer is affirmative, then society must satisfy the government's financial burden.

The myriad of mechanisms that patients must navigate to gain access to the healthcare system can be complex; many still require a gatekeeper system, a referral system for specialty care, and multiple networks of care, within or outside of a current system. Quality of care has become a huge issue in the last decade and has focused on entry-level education, science-based decision-making, and the avoidance of medical errors in practice.

As Americans live longer, technologies emerge, and leaders and healthcare providers find new ways to manage our healthcare system, the true measures noted above (i.e., cost, quality, and access) will persist. All stakeholders, including clinicians and their patients, will be required to learn to more efficiently and effectively manage the health of our citizens.

Cost (Affordability of Care)

According to the Henry J. Kaiser Family Foundation:

> The high and growing cost of health care is a significant issue for businesses, workers, and government. Spending on health care, which is a projected to be 18% of the US gross domestic product (GDP) in 2009, has consistently grown faster than the economy overall since the 1960s.[1]

The United States spends more on health care, both as a proportion of gross domestic product (GDP) and on a per-capita basis than any other nation in the world. Current estimates put US healthcare spending at approximately 18% of GDP, the world's highest, exceeding $2.3 billion in 2009. The health share of GDP is expected to continue its historic upward trend, projected to reach more than 30% of GDP by 2040.[2] The Kaiser Family Foundation & Health Research and Educational Trust reported:

> Employer-sponsored health insurance premiums have more than doubled in the last 9 years, a rate 4 times faster than cumulative wage increases. The United States spent approximately $2.2 trillion on health care in 2007, or an average of $7421 per person. This comes to 16.2% of GDP, nearly twice the average of other developed nations. Healthcare costs doubled from 1996 to 2006, and they are projected to rise to 25% of GDP in 2025 and to 49% in 2082. The proportion of spending attributable to Medicare and Medicaid in the healthcare system is expected to rise from 4% of GDP in 2007 to 19% of GDP in 2082, making it the principle driving force behind rising federal spending in the decades to come.[3]

The United States is the only major industrialized nation in the world lacking government-regulated or subsidized universal health care. In the United States, approximately 84% of citizens have health insurance, either through their employer (64%), purchased individually (9%), or provided by government programs (27%); with some overlap in these figures.[4] Other various publicly funded healthcare programs provide care for the elderly, disabled, children, veterans, and the poor. US government healthcare programs accounted for more than 44% of healthcare expenditures, making the US government the largest insurer in the nation.

It is also clear that health insurance is expensive; medical bills are overwhelmingly the most common reason for personal bankruptcy in the United States.[5] Without universal healthcare coverage of all American citizens, the healthcare system has evolved into a series of subsystems. Subsystems refer to components within the US health industry that are self-contained health services systems providing care to defined populations, such as the Veterans' Administration healthcare system.

Access to Care

Access to care typically refers to the ability of an individual to obtain medical care services in a timely, convenient, and affordable way. Access is a defining characteristic of the healthcare system, and in this instance the term is used in a policy context. In other instances, access means having health insurance, which in the US system is key to obtaining medical services. In the United States, individuals with access to health care are the following:

- Those with employer-based health insurance
- Those with private healthcare insurance
- Those covered under a government health program
- Those able to pay for their care

Access to care is measured by large-scale national surveys that include the National Health Interview Survey (NHIS), the National Ambulatory Medical Care Survey (NAMCS), and the Medical Expenditure Panel Survey (MEPS). These surveys are typically conducted by agencies such as the National Center for Health Statistics (a branch of the Centers for Disease Control [CDC]), the Health Resources and Services Administration (HRSA), or the CDC.

Quality of Care

In 2000, the Institute of Medicine report, *To Err Is Human*,[6] estimated that 100,000 Americans die each year from medication errors in hospitals. This staggering fact has taken hold in the public consciousness

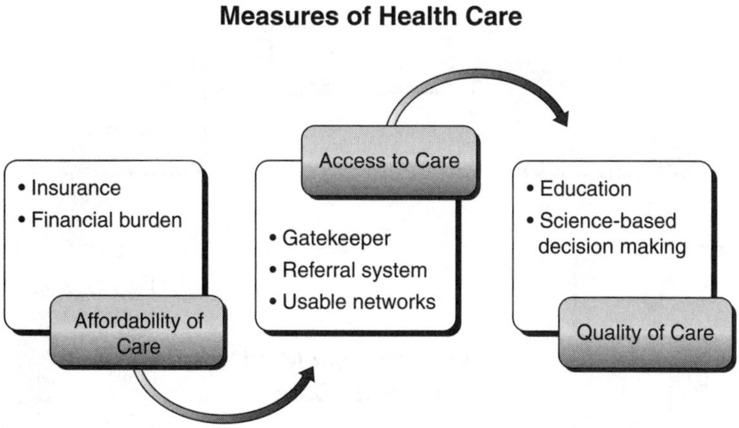

Measures of Health Care

Figure 1–1 Measures of Health Care

as emblematic of the problems with the quality of American health care (see **Figure 1-1**).

STAKEHOLDERS

It is important to recognize the groups or institutions that have a stake in how the healthcare system works in this country. The Department of Labor estimates that 13.6 million people are employed in the healthcare industry, approximately 10% of the workforce. Seven of the 20 fastest growing occupations are healthcare related. Between 2009 and 2016, the healthcare field will generate 3 million new jobs, more than any other industry[7] (see **Figure 1-2**).

Undoubtedly the largest and most impacted stakeholders are the patients. Multiple consumer organizations are monitoring patient rights. The next most impacted stakeholders are employers. Employers continue to be saddled with determining levels of healthcare coverage for their employees. A number of small and large organizations represent the rights of employers. The group that has the responsibility for providing healthcare, and the next group of stakeholders, is composed of providers. We will discuss this group in more detail later in the chapter. Hospitals and healthcare facilities

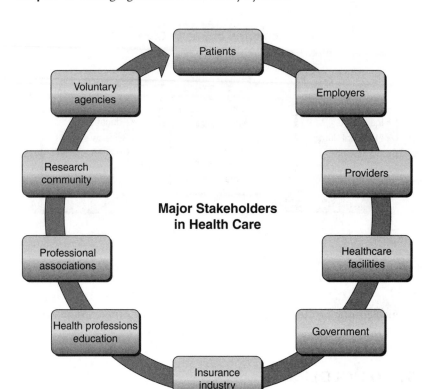

Figure 1–2 Healthcare Stakeholders

are the stakeholders at the very core of the healthcare system. These particular stakeholders have seen significant changes in the last decade regarding their overall role in health care. The government has become both a provider of and regulator of health care at both the state and federal levels, particularly with the creation of Medicare and Medicaid. Managed care organizations, preferred provider organizations (PPOs), and other insurers have been major stakeholders in healthcare delivery. Long-term care organizations have also become large stakeholders, particularly because Americans are living longer and thus are dealing with more multiple chronic illnesses. Voluntary and professional associations and agencies are also stakeholders, performing research and providing lobbying efforts. Another stakeholder are health professions' educational institutions. One cannot underestimate their importance in the present and future healthcare system in this country. We will discuss several of the major health professions in the healthcare system including physicians, nurse practitioners, and PAs.

Physicians

In the United States, the title physician is widely used and applies to any licensed physician. The term physician is used to describe those holding the degrees of Doctor of Medicine (MD) and Doctor of Osteopathic Medicine (DO). Beginning in the 19th century and accelerating in the 20th century, increasing urbanization and an emphasis on science and technology were factors that transformed medicine in America. Urbanization transformed US medical practice from a small-town cottage industry into a hospital-centered one. With breakthrough scientific discoveries, physicians became better equipped to treat and even cure diseases, and physicians became increasingly professionalized. Physicians concentrated their practices in urban areas, where they could see more patients and where they had better

Table 1–1 Clinicians in the United States

	Males	Females	Total	% of Total
Physicians (MD)[a]	665,647	256,257	921,904	77%
Physicians (DO)[b]	41,280	21,840	63,120	4%
Nurse Practitioners[c]	5,600	134,400	140,000	12%
Physician Assistants[d]	32,617	47,089	79,706	7%

[a]Physician Characteristics and Distribution in the U.S., 2008 Edition, American Medical Association.
[b]Available at: http://www.osteopathic.org/inside-aoa/about/who-we-are/Documents/Osteopathic-Medical-Profession-Report-2010.pdf Accessed January 8, 2011.
[c]Data derived from http://www.aanp.org/NR/rdonlyres/90C86114-C17C-407B-8056-D47956C9DB0F/0/AANPNPFactsLogo1111.pdf Accessed January 8, 2011.
[d]Available at: http://www.aapa.org/about-pas/data-and-statistics/aapa-census/2009-data. Accessed June, 2010.

access to hospitals that housed up-to-date diagnostic and therapeutic technologies.

There are 131 allopathic medical schools and 25 osteopathic medical schools in the United States. Medical education is typically at the tertiary level and is undertaken at a medical school approved by the Liaison Committee on Medical Education (LCME) sponsored by the Association of American Medical Colleges and the American Medical Association for MDs. The American Osteopathic Association's Commission on Osteopathic College Accreditation (COCA) currently accredits osteopathic medical schools. Depending on the university, entry to medical school may be directly from secondary school and/or may require prerequisite undergraduate education. Medical schools typically require undergraduate education (usually a 3- or 4-year degree, often in science) and are 4 or 5 years in length.

Physician Assistants

In the United States, a physician assistant (PA) is a clinician licensed to practice medicine with the supervision of a licensed physician. Physician assistants perform administrative and clinical tasks in hospitals and clinics with the supervision of physicians.

The PA profession began in the mid-1960s due to the shortage and maldistribution of primary care physicians in the United States. Eugene A. Stead of the Duke University Medical Center in North Carolina assembled the first class of PAs in 1965, composed of former US Navy hospital corpsmen. These individuals received considerable medical training during their military service and gained valuable experience during the Vietnam War. He based the curriculum of the PA program in part on his first-hand knowledge of the fast-track training of medical doctors during World War II.[8]

There are 146 accredited PA programs in the United States. The Accreditation Review Commission–Physician Assistants (ARC-PA), accredits PA programs. The majority are graduate programs leading to the award of master's degrees. Physician assistant education is based on the medical school model and is usually 2 to 3 years in duration. Unlike physicians, who must complete a minimum of three years of residency after completion of medical schools, PAs are not required to complete such residencies. Despite this, there are residency programs in several specialties for PAs who choose to continue formal education.

After graduation from an accredited PA program, PAs must pass the NCCPA-administered Physician Assistant National Certifying Exam (PANCE). This national certification is required for licensure in all states. To maintain certification, a PA must earn and log 100 hours of Continuing Medical Education (CME) every two years. A PA may also recertify every six years through successful completion of the Physician Assistant National Recertifying Exam (PANRE).

Nurse Practitioners

A nurse practitioner (NP) is a registered nurse who has completed advanced nursing education in the diagnosis and management of common and complex medical conditions. Like PAs, NPs provide a broad range of healthcare services. The American Academy of Nurse Practitioners defines nurse practitioners as licensed independent practitioners who practice in ambulatory, acute, and long-term care as primary and/or specialty care providers.[9] Nurse practitioners provide advanced nursing services to individuals, families, and groups according to their area of practice or specialty. As with all clinicians, NPs are licensed by the state in which they practice and are certified by a national board (usually through the American Nurses Credentialing Center or American Academy of Nurse Practitioners). These programs, offered by many universities with a School of Nursing, are graduate-level programs; upon successful completion, students may be awarded a Master of Science in Nursing (MSN) or Doctor of Nursing Practice (DNP) degree.

Before or after receiving state licensing, a nurse practitioner can apply for national certification from one of several professional nursing organizations such as the American Nurses Credentialing Center (ANCC) or the American Academy of Nurse Practitioners (AANP). Although it does not offer certification directly, the American Nurses Association (ANA) offers certification through its credentialing center, the ANCC. Some NPs pursue certification in a specialty. Several organizations oversee certification, including the following:

- American Association of Critical-Care Nurses
- American Psychiatric Nursing Association
- Board of Certification for Emergency Nursing
- Pediatric Nursing Certification Board
- National Certification Corporation for the Obstetric, Gynecologic, and Neonatal Nursing Specialties

CONCLUSION

The US healthcare delivery system is undergoing a transformation. It is possible that by the end of 2011, the system may see modifications that provide health insurance coverage for a significant portion of the population of Americans that currently lack health coverage.

Demographics are shifting in ways unexpected only a few years ago. The aging of America will alter society, with 1 in 5 individuals being retired by 2030. This factor will significantly influence the labor force, the economy, and will strain employment-intensive services such as health care, transportation, and food services. Medicare, the US healthcare entitlement for the elderly, will not be adequate to meet demand, and few good ideas have been promoted to address this shortfall. More years in retirement may diminish resources for children and working adults. Special pressures on the elderly will emerge in areas where they are concentrated, such as Arizona, Nevada, and Florida. Forecasting the changing picture of healthcare financing necessitates understanding policy changes at federal and state/provincial levels and movements in the employer and consumer markets. It also requires tracking shifts in demographics and technology. Changes, underway for some time, reveal government's priorities to expand medical coverage for more Americans. It is likely that some healthcare reform will occur in this country and experts acknowledge that any such measure will necessarily include a workforce component. These policy changes will increase demand on a healthcare system that is struggling with labor costs. PAs and NPs offer an opportunity to provide this care at less expensive salaries. The substitutability of these providers for traditional physician services could indicate that they are likely to be used in more ways to help fill the gaps in the demand for healthcare access and services.

Most believe that in 2011, the US healthcare system is on an unsustainable path. Expenditures as a share of GDP are already substantially higher than in other developed countries, and they are projected to grow rapidly in the next 30 years. This growth threatens to have a devastating impact on workers' take-home pay and the government's budget deficit. The number of Americans without health insurance is likely to increase from its already very high level and thus undermine the health of the population. If it can be accomplished, healthcare reform may slow the growth rate of healthcare costs, maintain choices of doctors and health plans, and expand coverage. Healthcare reform could have major benefits for the US economy.

REFERENCES

1. Kaiser Family Foundation. *Your Resource for Health Policy Information, Research, and Analysis.* March, 2009. Available at: http://www.kff.org. Accessed November 30, 2010.
2. US Department of Health and Human Services. Centers for Medicare and Medicaid Services. National Health Expenditure Accounts. *National Health Expenditure Projections 2008–2018.* Available at: http://www.cms .hhs.gov/NationalHealthExpendData/downloads/proj2008.pdf. Accessed November 30, 2010.
3. Kaiser Family Foundation and Health Research and Educational Trust. *Employer Health Benefits 2008 Annual Survey.* Menlo Park, CA: Kaiser Family Foundation; 2008. Available at: http://ehbs.kff.org/? page=abstract&id=1. Accessed November 30, 2010.
4. Shi L, Singh DA. *Delivering Health Care in America: A Systems Approach.* 4th ed. Boston, MA: Jones & Bartlett; 2008.
5. Himmelstein DU, Warren E, Thorne D, Woolhandler S. Illness and injury as contributors to bankruptcy. *Health Affairs,* 2005, W563-W573. Available at: http://content.healthaffairs.org/content/early/2005/02/02/hlthaff .w5.63. Accessed March 30, 2009.
6. Institute of Medicine. *To Err Is Human: Building a Safer Health System.* Washington, DC: National Academies Press; 2000.

7. US Department of Labor, Bureau of Labor Statistics Web site. Available at: http://www.bls.gov. Accessed January 12, 2009.
8. American Academy of Physician Assistants Web site. Available at: http://www.certphysicianassistant.com/aapa-php? Accessed November 30, 2010.
9. American Academy of Nurse Practitioners Web site. Available at: http://www.aanp.org/AANPCMS2. Accessed November 30, 2010.

Chapter 2

Demographics of the Physician Assistant Profession

At this writing, there are nearly 80,000 clinically practicing physician assistants (PAs) in the United States. These PAs see an average of 92 patients a week, 460 patients a month, and 4600 patients per year. With a reported 93% of all PAs practicing clinically, that translates into over 370 million patient visits per year to PAs, or 1 million patients taken care of each day by PAs. These patients are seen in primary care clinics, medical specialty practices, hospitals, emergency rooms, and a myriad of other practice settings.[1]

Would Eugene A. Stead, MD, considered the founder of the PA profession, and his colleagues in the early 1960s have envisioned today's demographic profile of the PA profession? There are currently 146 accredited PA educational programs across the country and the number is rising; most are affiliated with medical schools and universities.[2] This number contrasts with the reported 131 allopathic medical schools and 25 osteopathic medical schools. Dr. Stead's crystal ball probably did not contemplate today's 12,000 PA students and nearly 6000 annual graduates. They might not have anticipated that the number of practicing PAs would increase by 50,000 between

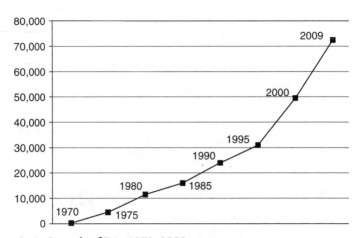

Figure 2–1 Growth of PAs 1970–2009

Source: Data from AAPA 2009, National Physician Assistant Census Report. Available at: http://www.aapa.org/images/stories/Data_2009/National_Final_with_Graphics.pdf. Accessed January 8, 2011.

1991 and 2007 and that, during a 5-year period from 1992 to 1997, the total number of graduates from nonphysician clinician training programs (PA and nurse practitioner) would more than double[3] (see **Figure 2-1**).

Based on the 2009 American Academy of Physician Assistants census, 65.2% of PA respondents were female and 11.6% were minority (non-white). The mean age of census responders was 41 years. It is important to note that 93% of PA respondents stated that they were in clinical practice, while 4% report working as PA educators. While 88% of respondents reported working in one clinical setting, 12% work multiple clinical jobs. Only 9% of respondents worked in the government sector; the Department of Veterans Affairs is the largest government employer of PAs. Interestingly, 37.5% of respondents to the census report their primary work setting to be in a hospital—most commonly inpatient units, emergency rooms, and hospital outpatient units (see **Figure 2-2**). The mean age of all respondents was 41 years, with a mean age at time of graduation from PA school of 30 years of age. The mean time span in clinical practice was 10.1 years, with a

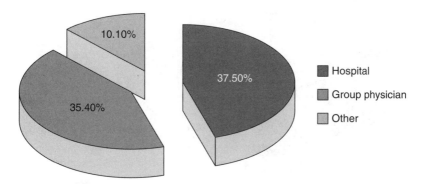

Figure 2–2 PA Practice Settings
Source: Data from AAPA 2009, National Physician Assistant Census Report. Available at: http://www.aapa.org/images/stories/Data_2009/National_Final_with_Graphics.pdf. Accessed January 8, 2011.

mean of 7.1 years in their current specialty. Only 15% of respondent PAs were working in rural areas.[1]

As are physicians, new PA graduates are leaning more frequently toward specialty PA practice (see Chapter 3). Today nearly two-thirds of graduates are working in non-primary care disciplines (and trends show that PAs, especially female graduates, are shunning rural practice).[1] Physician assistants practice in more than 60 specialty fields; 35.7% reported their specialty as one of the primary care fields (see **Figure 2-3**). Interestingly, Druss et al.,[4] in their comparison study, found that the number of patients receiving acute medical care from physicians has remained stable, while acute care from nonphysician clinicians declined by 28% between 1987 and 1997, indicating a move by nonphysician clinicians (NPCs) into chronic and preventive care. Multiple models have shown a high quality of care for patients with chronic conditions when cared for by NPCs. From 1987 to 1997 the proportion of patients who saw NPCs rose from 23.5% to 30.9%. An interesting finding in the Druss study was more NPCs were working at the same location as a physician in 1997 (41.1%) compared to 1987 (14.3%). This is another indicator of NPC movement into specialty practice.[4]

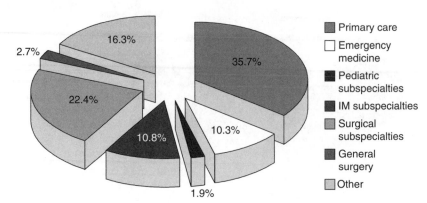

Figure 2–3 PA Specialties

Source: Data from AAPA 2009, National Physician Assistant Census Report. Available at: http://www.aapa.org/images/stories/Data_2009/National_Final_with_Graphics.pdf. Accessed January 8, 2011.

Physician assistants have reached the recognition of a well-established health profession, with licensure in all states and the District of Columbia. They have prescribing authority in all states and commissioned officer status in all branches of the uniformed services. Physician assistant services are reimbursed by Medicare, Medicaid, and the majority third-party payers.

Physician assistant utilization for inpatient services has gained increasing attention since 2003 as hospitals have adjusted to General Medical Education (GME) work-hour limitations.[4] It is also true that PAs provide a full range of inpatient services with no decline in the quality of care while providing an element of continuity to care.[5]

PAs play a huge role in the federal healthcare system. More than 3000 PAs provide care to federal employees within the Department of Veterans Affairs, the Public Health Services, and the US Military. According to Hooker, "as of 2008, ~1300 PAs serve on land or sea or in the air, with many in special hardship situations. In addition, >400 civilian PAs serve in the Ready Reserves and National Guard in 50 states and 4 territories."[6]

The success of the PA profession can be measured by economic analysis (see Chapter 5), by the steady growth of new training programs, by an incredible number of interested applicants, by graduate productivity, and by the relatively short time span that has passed since a handful of ex-medics accepted the opportunity to pioneer a profession.

However, the ultimate measure of the PA profession is not production or cost ratios; it is not demographic trends or numbers. The ultimate measure is this: Do PAs provide services that meet the medical needs of the patient in a productive and complementary fashion with their supervising physician? Nearly half a century of data indicates high patient satisfaction—professional success.

REFERENCES

1. 2009 American Academy of Physician Assistants census. Available at: http://www.aapa.org/about-pas/data-and-statistics/aapa-2009. Accessed November 30, 2010.
2. Physician Assistants Education Association census/2009-data accessed at PAEA Web site. Available at: http://www.paeaonline.org/index .php?ht=d/sp/i/206/pid/206. Accessed March 1, 2010.
3. Liang M. *Twenty-Fifth Annual Report on Physician Assistant Educational Programs in the United States: 2008–2009*. Alexandria, VA: PAEA; June, 2010.
4. Druss BG, Marcus SC, Gifson M, Tandielan T, Pincus HA. Trends in healthcare by nonphysician clinicians in the United States. *N Engl J Med.* 2003;348:130–137.
5. Duffy K. Physician assistants: Filling the gap in patient care in academic hospitals. *Perspect Phys Assist Educ.* 2003;14(3):158–167.
6. Hooker RS. Federally employed physician assistants. *Mil Med.* 2008;173(9):895–899.

Chapter 3

Growing Physician Assistant Specialization

Medical specialization in the United States is not a new concept. In fact, medical specialization began in the 19th century. In the 1880s, specialization came to be viewed as a necessity because clinical researchers were forced to "specialize" or focus on a particular area to expand medical knowledge. This need was compounded by the belief that large populations could be best managed through proper classification.[1] The increasing scope of surgery contributed to the specialization trend. Admittedly, most general surgeons had a special interest, and for a long time there had been an element of specialization in such fields as ophthalmology, orthopedics, obstetrics, and gynecology. Before long it became apparent that, to achieve progress in certain areas, surgeons would have to concentrate their attention on that particular classification of human disease. In turn, as teaching hospitals became more specialized, general hospitals became more involved in providing general clinical training to medical students.

The American Board of Medical Specialties (ABMS), created in 1933, is a not-for-profit national organization. It currently reports 24 approved medical specialty boards that have developed standards in the ongoing evaluation and certification of physicians.[2] The ABMS is recognized as the "gold standard" in physician certification.

The current recognized medical specialties and the years they were created are listed in **Table 3-1**. In recent years, the issue of physician assistant (PA) specialty practice has come to the forefront of the field, although its current prominence in profession-wide discussion should not be taken to mean the present conversation is the first iteration of this discussion in the PA community. In fact, this debate is in some ways nearly as old as the profession itself. In the profession's early days, "specialties" were identified as the difference between primary care and surgery, but even those conversations often occurred under the banner of PA specialization.

Presently, among the more than 70,000 PAs in clinical practice in the United States, more than 65% are working in a specialty setting[3] (see **Table 3-2**). Even though the American Academy of Physician Assistants (AAPA) estimates that PAs practice in over 60 different specialty fields, these estimates are often confounded because it is difficult to determine whether the PA is actually performing specialty tasks and procedures or performing primary care in a specialty practice.

Table 3-1 ABMS Recognized Medical Specialties

1. Allergy and Immunology (1971)	14. Otolaryngology (1933)
2. Anesthesiology (1941)	15. Pathology (1936)
3. Colon and Rectal Surgery (1949)	16. Pediatrics (1935)
4. Dermatology (1933)	17. Physical Medicine and Rehabilitation (1947)
5. Emergency Medicine (1979)	
6. Family Medicine (1969)	18. Plastic Surgery (1941)
7. Internal Medicine (1936)	19. Preventive Medicine (1949)
8. Medical Genetics (1991)	20. Psychiatry and Neurology (1935)
9. Neurological Surgery (1940)	
10. Nuclear Medicine (1971)	21. Radiology (1935)
11. Obstetrics and Gynecology (1933)	22. Surgery (1937)
12. Ophthalmology (1933)	23. Thoracic Surgery (1971)
13. Orthopedic Surgery (1935)	24. Urology (1935)

Source: Data from the American Board of Medical Specialities. Available at: http://www.abms.org/About_ABMS/who_we_are.aspx. Accessed January 8, 2011.

As greater numbers of PAs move into areas of specialty practice, many will seek membership in a specialty organization. Currently, there are 24 recognized specialty organizations by the AAPA. **Table 3-3** shows the names and Web sites for contact information.

The trend toward specialization within the PA community has, nonetheless, created opportunities for clinicians practicing in those areas to seek recognition of their proficiency.[4] To address these issues the National Commission on Certification of Physician Assistants (NCCPA), whose mission is to assure that certified PAs meet professional standards of knowledge and skills, began to develop mechanisms for specialty recognition in 2006.

It is well known and demonstrated that PA practice ranges from primary care to specialty and subspecialty services, with all care being provided with physician supervision. Thus, in order to fulfill its mission, the NCCPA has developed appropriate eligibility criteria and assessment mechanisms for Certificates of Added Qualification

Table 3–2 Percent Distribution of Clinically Practicing PAs by General Specialty in 2007

Specialty	% of Total
Family/general medicine	24.9%
General internal medicine	6.9%
Emergency medicine	10.3%
Pediatrics	2.4%
Surgery	2.7%
Internal med subspecialties	11.3%
Pediatric subspecialties	1.6%
Surgical subspecialties	22.2%
Obstetrics & gynecology	2.4%
Occupational medicine	2.4%
Other	12.8%

Source: Data from AAPA 2009, National Physician Assistant Census Report. Available at: http://www.aapa.org/images/stories/Data_2009/National_Final_with_Graphics.pdf. Accessed January 8, 2011.

Table 3–3 Recognized Specialty Organizations for PAs

Specialty	Name	Contact Information
Nephrology	American Academy of Nephrology PAs	http://www.aanpa.org/
Occupational Medicine	American Academy of PAs in Occupational Medicine	http://www.aapaoccmed.org
Allergy, Asthma, & Immunology	American Academy of PAs in Allergy, Asthma, and Immunology	http://www.aapa-aai.com/
Surgery	American Association of Surgical PAs	http://www.aaspa.com/
Endocrine	American Society of Endocrine PAs	http://www.endocrine-pa.com/
Family Practice	Association of Family Practice PAs	http://www.afppa.org/
Neurosurgical	Association of Neurosurgical PAs	http://www.anspa.org/
Cardiology	Association of PAs in Cardiology	http://cardiologypa.org/
Cardiovascular Surgery	Association of PAs in Cardiovascular Surgery	http://www.apacvs.org/
Obstetrics & Gynecology	Association of PA's in Obstetrics & Gynecology	http://www.paobgyn.org/
Oncology	Association of PAs in Oncology	http://apao.cc/
Anesthesia	Association of PAs in Anesthesia	http://www.paanesthesiaworld.us/
Plastic Surgery	Association of Plastic Surgery PAs	http://www.apspa.net/new/
Gastroenterology	Gastroenterology PAs	http://www.gipas.org/
Orthopedic Surgery	PAs in Orthopedic Surgery	http://www.paos.org/
Psychiatry	PAs in Psychiatry	http://www.psychpa.com/
Pediatrics	Society of PAs in Pediatrics	http://www.spaponline.org/
Dermatology	Society of Dermatology PAs	http://www.dermpa.org/

Table 3–3 Recognized Specialty Organizations for PAs (*Continued*)

Specialty	Name	Contact Information
Emergency Medicine	Society of Emergency Medicine PAs	http://www.sempa.org/default.asp
Geriatrics	Society of PAs Caring for the Elderly	http://www.geri-pa.org/
Addiction	Society of PAs in Addiction Medicine	Contact: Bernard Stuetz, MA, PA-C, bjspaethic@aol.com
Otorhinolaryngology/ Head & Neck	Society of PAs in Otorhinolaryngology/ Head & Neck Surgery	http://www.entpa.org/
Rheumatology	Society of PAs in Rheumatology	http://www.rheumpas.org/
Urology	Urological Association of PAs	http://www.uapanet.org/

Source: Data from AAPA 2009, National Physician Assistant Census Report. Available at: http://www.aapa.org/images/stories/Data_2009/National_Final_with_Graphics.pdf. Accessed January 8, 2011.

(CAQ). Like all current NCCPA programs, CAQ is a competency-based program.

In addition to the Institute of Medicine (IOM), employers, regulatory boards, and patient advocate groups are placing heightened emphasis on patient safety and risk management. There are additional concerns that the complexities and increasing demands of healthcare practice are placing constraints and increased burdens on the supervisory aspects of the physician–PA relationship. The profession's growth and increasing visibility has resulted in the need for greater accountability.

The CAQ, voluntary and independent of NCCPA's certification and recertification processes, is guided by a few key premises. The CAQ supports and reinforces relationships between specialty PAs and physicians, and it supports the credentialing process while avoiding the creation of barriers to licensure and practice.

To qualify for a specialty CAQ, PAs must first satisfy two basic prerequisites: (1) current PA certification and (2) possession of a valid, unrestricted license to practice as a PA in at least one jurisdiction in the United States or its territories, or unrestricted privileges to practice as a PA for a government agency. (Note: If a PA holds licenses in multiple states, all of the licenses must be unrestricted.)

For PAs meeting those basic prerequisites, the CAQ process includes four core requirements: (1) Category I specialty CME, (2) 1 to 2 years of experience, (3) procedural and patient experience appropriate for the specialty, and (4) a specialty exam.

The first three core requirements may be completed in any order. Once those are complete, PAs are eligible for the exam. More CAQ programs for physician assistants in emergency medicine, orthopedic surgery, cardiovascular surgery, nephrology, and psychiatry are scheduled to launch in late 2011.

Both PAs and physician specialists along with specialty organizations assisted in the development of the specialty-specific requirements through advisory committees that (1) further defined the CME, (2) logged procedures and patient cases, and (3) established experience requirements for each specialty.

Thus, the movement of PAs into CAQs is a fairly new phenomenon that should be monitored to identify trends, postgraduate education needs, and potential barriers to moving between specialties.

REFERENCES

1. Weiz G. Bulletin of the History of Medicine. *Hist Med.* 2003;77:563–575.
2. American Board of Medical Specialties. Available at: http://www.abms.org/About_ABMS/who_we_are.aspx. Accessed November 30, 2010.
3. American Academy of Physician Assistants. Available at: http://www.aapa.org/about-pas/data-and-statistics/aapa-census/2009-data. Accessed November 30, 2009.
4. Cawley J. A lull before the storm? Expect to hear more about PA specialty certification. *Advance for PAs.* Available at: http://physician-assistant.advanceweb.com/Editorial/Content/Editorial.aspx?CC=123399. Accessed November 30, 2009.

Chapter 4

International Development

Although the physician assistant (PA) "concept" is often considered to be a US development, similar health workforce strategies have been utilized throughout the world—both historically and currently.[1] Just as the US PA and nurse practitioner (NP) movements arose from rapid US social change in the post-Vietnam era, similar new types of clinicians developed simultaneously in other countries.

According to a conversation with Ruth Ballweg, Associate Professor at the University of Washington, following a number of professional trips to Africa (March 2010), after 1950 in Africa, political conflict, the rejection of European colonialism, the development of independent governments, and the mass exodus of African physicians led to restructuring of the health workforce. In Mozambique, for example, where over 20 million people are cared for by less than 700 physicians, a new profession of "technicos" was developed in the mid-1970s to deliver primary care and to perform specific tasks such as caesarian sections. In Lesotho, a program developed by Dr. Richard Smith trained MEDEX (MED = medical, EX = Extension, i.e. extension of the physician) whose services became the foundation of health care in the small country. With the occurrence and spread of HIV/AIDS—and the continued exodus of African physicians from

African countries—nonphysician clinicians (NPCs) have become a major component of health workforce strategies.

Dr. Fitzhugh Mullan and Dr. Seble Frehywot described Africa's NPCs in 2007 in *The Lancet*.[2] Surveying health workers in 25 of the 47 countries in sub-Saharan Africa, they found that NPCs exceeded the number of physicians in 9 countries. There was no standardization of training or roles across these 25 countries, although the training programs could be divided into those that gave additional training to nurses and those that chose non-nurses as students. Overall, the NPCs training was practical and often specific to local and indigenous disorders. Often recruited from rural and poor areas, these NPCs were more likely to remain in their home communities than physicians and nurses.

The "brain drain" continues to have its largest impact on Africa. In 2004, Hagopian et al from the University of Washington described and measured the African brain drain—and the concern in African countries about this issue:

> African governments have been very clear about their objections to the wholesale migration of their physicians to rich countries. In 1996, South Africa's then-Deputy President Thabo Mbeki implored the World Health Assembly to take measures to stop the flow of physicians from poor countries to rich ones. Nonetheless, large numbers of Africa-trained physicians leave home upon completion of their medical school training in search of careers in higher-income countries. They leave behind health systems in sub-Saharan Africa that are severely stressed: life expectancy is only 50 years. 162 children in 1000 die before reaching their fifth birthdays, and only half have access to clean water sources. Further, AIDS prevalence among those 15 to 49 years old is estimated to be 8.4% and in four countries, adult HIV prevalence exceeds 30%.[3]

Globally, a number of new healthcare worker programs were the product of MEDEX International, created by Dr. Richard Smith at the University of Hawaii. (Dr. Smith had originally founded the MEDEX Northwest Physician Assistant Program at the University of Washington). Dr. Smith and his team developed a technology to train mid-level health workers, which was implemented globally in five countries. The MEDEX technology included a series of clinical modules that could be used for either training or clinical practice.

The MEDEX project was developed and facilitated by teams of clinicians, educators, and trainers, including representatives of the host countries. A key feature of the MEDEX series was a design that allowed each individual country, or delivery system, to "adapt" the materials and training to the needs of the specific country or region. The idea of "adapting" versus "adopting" a new clinical role has emerged as an important component of the evolving global discussion about defining PAs, or "physician-assistant-like" clinicians and what that means in terms of education, clinical training, regulation, and supervision.[4]

The MEDEX systems-based model for healthcare workforce development includes a series of steps to be taken in creating a new healthcare profession. Those steps include the following:

1. The collaborative model: involving stakeholders and communities.
2. The "receptive framework": creating infrastructure such as regulation, funding, and reimbursement strategies for the new career parallel to the development of initial training programs.
3. Competency-based training: deciding what the new health workers should do and building specific, focused curriculum around those needs compared to nonspecific basic science training preceding generic clinical training.
4. Practitioner involvement (supervision): involving senior clinicians in planning and supervision.
5. Structured/planned deployment: choosing students from the neediest communities and assuring that they are trained, employed, and retained there.
6. Continuing medical education: assuring dynamic practice through ongoing building of knowledge and skills.[5]

Dr. Smith's MEDEX premise was that the development of new healthcare roles involved not just curricular design but also the creation of a stakeholder infrastructure to support the new career. New PA programs developing globally illustrate the importance of these steps.

The Netherlands has been the first European nation to develop the PA role. Spenkelink-Schut et al. described the country's need for PAs in the *Journal of Physician Assistant Education*:

> In The Netherlands there is a growing shortage of adequately trained health care workers, an increasing demand for medical services, a growing political pressure to contain the costs of health care, a shift from hospital care to outpatient care and from curative care to preventive care and increased demand to apply emerging biomedical technologies in health care. The concept of "demand-driven care"—a concept that empowers the patient in the coordination and organization of health care—plays a key role in the modernization of the Dutch health care system and forms an instrument to liberalize public activities.[6]

The Netherlands was concerned specifically about efficiencies in the healthcare system and the redistribution of tasks from "highly educated and relatively expensive physicians" to others. The University of Utrecht first developed a cardiovascular surgery role for PAs with subsequent movement into primary care and other specialties.

Physician delegation and supervision are key features of the PA model in The Netherlands:

> The curriculum pays specific attention to the delegation of tasks from physicians to the PA. Medical supervisors of trainees should be able to decide when a trainee may be trusted to bear responsibility to perform a professional medical activity, given the level of competence he or she has reached. This services both education and patient care. In this respect, trust is essential. The PA should be able to clearly indicate the limits of his/her ability, should have an active learning attitude, possess social skills, and contribute to the supply-chain process in health care. ... The extent of the medical care that the PA provides is restricted by (1) agreements on delegation of tasks as agreed between the supervising physician and the PA, (2) the limited medical competence of the PA compared with that of physicians.[6]

By 2008 the number of PA programs in The Netherlands had grown to 5, with 271 students enrolled and 194 PAs in practice.[6]

Commonwealth countries also moved to create PA programs using pilot programs to demonstrate the utilization and acceptability of the new role. The first pilot program, in the United Kingdom, placed US PAs in a variety of primary care and emergency room settings. An interim report of the project by Woodin et al. at the University of

Birmingham had some "first impressions" that helped to move the PA profession forward in the United Kingdom.[7]

Anecdotally, the PA role has been well received by colleagues. Factors facilitating this integration included a teamwork ethos, which is a fundamental characteristic of the PA role and training, and the induction period with the supervising physician, which continued until the point at which both general practitioners (GP) and PA had established understanding of, and confidence in, each other's practice.

A further facilitating factor was the flexibility of the PA role. Evidence of this was provided not only by the range of conditions seen, but also by the reports of PAs taking on some work normally undertaken by nursing staff to help cover tasks during vacancy periods. PAs have also undertaken home visits, have run clinics, and have provided service to a residential home. Furthermore, there has been discussion of potential for involvement in off-hours work, and minor surgery.

Patients appear to have responded well to the role, with no adverse reactions and with evidence of satisfaction from repeat visits and anecdotal comments. The only, and limited, reported complaints have related to having to wait for a prescription.

There is little evidence in this study that the introduction of the PA role has resulted in redefinition of the general practitioner (GP, family doctor) or other professional roles, re-profiling of work or professional boundaries, or significant service development or service improvement, other than improved access times. The main impact to date has been to increase the capacity of the primary care workforce to deal with routine work, in an area where GPs are difficult to recruit.[7]

The *Journal of the Association of Physician Assistant Education* reviewed the progress of the UK PA programs in an article by Begg et al.:

> A decade since the first American PAs were successfully recruited, the UK is starting to produce its own. The first homegrown graduates (20) are in practice and four PA programs are in place, with more than 50 students in training. A further 100 are expected to start their training in 2009.
> ...we believe the value of the role for health care in the UK is now beyond discussion.[8]

Ultimately a stakeholder's process in the United Kingdom developed the Competence and Curriculum Framework for Physician Assistant Programs and defined the PA role with supervision as a key feature:

> (A) new healthcare professional who, while not a doctor, works to the medical model, with the attitudes, skills and knowledge based to deliver holistic care and treatment within the general medicine and/or general practice team under defined levels of supervision.[9]

A pilot project was created in Scotland that, in 2006–2008, placed 15 US-trained PAs in primary care, emergency medicine, off-hours clinics, intermediate care, an acute receiving unit, and orthopedics. A detailed evaluation reported overall positive outcomes, although the PAs generally felt underutilized, partially because they did not have prescriptive privileges. Supervision was also an issue, with a wide range of expectations and/or experiences between supervising physicians and PAs: some oversupervised and some provided inconsistent levels of supervision. As a result, the designs of subsequent pilots in other countries were more proactive in providing explicit directives, training, and evaluation for supervision.

The Scottish evaluation team, led by Jane Farmer, commented on global PA development:

> The current wave of international development in deploying and training PAs can ... be viewed in alternative ways. Firstly, it could be viewed as a 'fashion.' The PA profession is neatly packaged, emanates from the USA (as many health system 'fashions' do), has some assiduous 'product champions' and is 'promoted' in a panacea-like way. Alternatively PAs can be viewed as THE profession, designed as uniquely adaptable, that is moving from the USA to other parts of the world at this time expressly because it can meet the world's current health workforce gaps. In the USA it fills the gaps for primary care generalists, secondary care registrars (in the wake of working time changes) and feeds the HMO system by taking care of routine medical work. In non-metropolitan areas of Canada, Australia and the developing world it supplies generalist medical staff where it is difficult to recruit. England has experienced gaps in primary care in disadvantaged areas and is experiencing the same gaps as Scotland in secondary care thrown up by changes in doctor's training and European Union working time legislation. As in other countries there is likely to be an inevitable level of resistance to PAs from

established professions... It was significant, in this evaluation, that many medical and nursing professionals who started with skepticism about PAs, changed to enthusiasts who recognized the potential in the PA role once they had worked with PAs.[10]

Meanwhile Canada, which had had PAs only in its military forces, explored the utilization of PAs through a large emergency-room-based pilot program in Ontario. The Ontario program became controversial when the decision was made to include International Medical Graduates (IMGs).

The selected IMGs, all of whom were eligible for the relatively few positions in physician residency training programs, were "socialized" to the PA role in a 4-month program. Central to this orientation program was the concept of being a supervised professional in contrast to being an independent professional.

The Ottawa pilot addressed the supervision role by acknowledging that the scope of practice of each PA should be built on the supervising physician's assessment of the individual PA's competencies, skills, and experience in a specific type of practice setting. Physicians provided feedback that established specific guidelines for PA supervision. The guidelines subsequently developed in consultation with regulators recommended the following:

- The primary supervising physician assesses the PA's skills and abilities before the PA begins to practice as part of the team.
- The supervising physician initially provides direct supervision of any clinical assessment or care provided by the PA.
- The physician determines when a PA may work without direct supervision (less-structured supervision still required).[11]

The final evaluation of the Ottawa project was positive—particularly in the areas of more efficient "throughput" and decreased waiting time for patients. As a result, Ontario committed to providing funding to extend the emergency room project for two more years. Nevertheless, physicians still felt that the main challenge of the project was "a lack of formal orientation/training process for the supervising physician and the PA."[12]

Canada moved ahead with the creation of new civilian PA programs. In September 2009, new programs opened at McMaster University in Ontario and at the University of Manitoba in Winnipeg. In addition, the province of Ontario has supported the development of a PA program at the University of Toronto and its affiliated campuses. Presently, in British Columbia a Ministry of Health steering committee is considering an additional pilot project to examine previously unevaluated clinical roles.

Australia has also been interested in using PAs to address the problems of physician shortages and maldistribution. Ironically the interest in PAs and NPs has continued despite a countrywide decision to double the size of medical school entry classes. Two PA pilot projects began in 2009. South Australia's small pilot project was designed to demonstrate the utilization of PAs in specialty surgical roles (GI surgery and anesthesia) and pediatrics. Queensland's Ministry of Health created a PA pilot program to address rural health needs as well as inpatient cardiology roles. In Queensland, these 1-year programs were designed as "prologues" to the development of new PA programs at the University of Queensland and James Cook University.

Learning from the other Commonwealth pilot projects, the Queensland program has included formal training in PA supervision for physicians by the medical director of a US PA training program and videotaping that training for future use.

Moving ahead without a pilot project, the South African National Department of Health mandated the creation of PAs (called "clinical associates") in each of the nation's seven medical schools. By 2009, three had created new programs: University of Pretoria, University of Walter Sisulu, and the University of Witswatersrand. In August 2008, Manto Tshabalala-Msimang, then the South Africa Minister of Health, described the process and the expectations for the new clinical associates:

> Consensus was reached that at the end of the training of Clinical Associates, they will be a competent, professional member of the health care team with the necessary knowledge, skills and attitudes to function effectively in the district health system in South Africa, primarily working with and under the supervision of a qualified medical practitioner.

The clinical associate's practice will include medical services within the education, training and experience of the clinical associate delegated by the supervising doctor.

Clinical Associates will be permitted to provide any medical service delegated to them by the supervising registered medical practitioner when such service is within their scope of practice, forms a component of the doctor's scope of practice, and is provided with supervision by a doctor. The clinical associate will thus be considered the agent of their supervising doctors in the performance of all practice-related activities including the ordering of diagnostic, therapeutic, and other medical services.[13]

A common thread for global PA program development is the issue of supervision. In developing countries, the brain drain for physicians may lead to inadequate numbers of physicians remaining to provide direct care, much less to provide supervision and support. These settings may actually develop innovations in supervision using new—but basic—technologies such as cell phones with cameras, and video Internet. These "developed countries"—with broad scopes for PA practice—and the expectation of complex decision-making, must continue to pay attention to the issue of physician supervision for practicing PAs. This definition of supervision includes support for the role and the individual PA, planning for the acquisition of new knowledge and/or skill sets, concurrent availability for consultation, and retrospective quality activities such as selective chart review and outcome oversight. Significantly, many skills for supervising PAs are also applicable to emerging team-based practice models.

REFERENCES

1. Ballweg R. History of the Profession. In: Ballweg R, Stolberg S, Sullivan E, eds. *Physician Assistant: A Guide to Clinical Practice.* 4th ed. Philadelphia, PA: Saunders/Elsevier; 2008:1.
2. Mullan F, Frehywot S. Non-physician clinicians in 47 sub-saharan African countries. *The Lancet.* 2007;370(9605):2158–2163.
3. Hagopian A, Thompson MJ, Fordyce M, Johnson K, Hart G. The migration of physicians from sub-Saharan Africa to the United States of America: measures of the African brain drain. *Human Resources for Health 2004*, p. 2. Available at: http://www.human-resources-health.com/content/2/1/17. Accessed November 30, 2010.

4. Personal communication with Richard Smith, MD, July 2009.

5. MEDEX Northwest Division of Physician Assistant Studies Physician Assistant Training Program. *The MEDEX Demonstration Program.* A Report for Department of Health Services, University of Washington School of Public Health and Community Medicine and the School of Medicine. Seattle, WA. Vol I, 1971.

6. Spenkelink-Schut G, Cate O, Helianthe S, Kort H. Training the physician assistant in The Netherlands. *PAEA Journal.* 2008;19(4)46–53.

7. Woodin J, McLeod H, McManus R. *The Introduction of US-trained Physician Assistants to primary care in Tipton: First impressions.* Birmingham, UK: Health Services Management Centre, University of Birmingham; 2004.

8. Begg P, Ross N, Parle J. Physician assistant education in the United Kingdom: The first five years. *Journal of the Association of Physician Assistant Programs.* 2008;19(3):47–50.

9. Black N, Rafferty AM, West E, Gough P. Health care workforce research: Identifying the agenda. *J Health Serv Res & Policy.* 2004;9(suppl 1):62–64.

10. Farmer J, Currie M, West C, Hyman J, Arnot N. *Evaluation of Physician Assistants To NHS Scotland, Final Report.* Edinburgh, Scotland: UHA Millennium Institute; 2009;4.6:41.

11. Mikhael N, Ozon P, Rhule C. *Defining the Physician Assistant Role in Ontario: Ontario Physician Assistant Scope of Practice Statement and Ontario Physician Assistant Competency Profile,* MOHLTC, OMA, 2007. Available at: http://www.cpso.on./ca/Policies/delegation.htm. Accessed March 30, 2009.

12. Ministry of Health and Long Term Care. *Introducing Physician Assistants in Ontario,* Ottawa, Canada: HealthForceOntario; 2008.

13. Tshabalala-Msimang M. Speech given by South African Minister of Health, Official Launch of the Clinical Programme in South Africa, 2008.

Chapter 5

Physician Assistant Economics

Healthcare cost for the American economy is greater than 16% of the gross domestic product (GDP) and is rising alarmingly.[1,2] Current studies suggest there is a physician shortage without a workable short-term solution through 2015, especially in primary care.[3] The role for the physician assistant (PA) remains favorable, and the passage of the new Health Care Affordability Act (HCAA), further improves the role of the PA.[4] The HCAA is important for the PA and the supervising physician for 2 reasons. First it includes pro-PA language that empowers the physician–PA healthcare delivery model. Second, a significant portion of the program's funding is derived through cost savings in payment for healthcare services that the physician–PA model could favorably impact (HR 3590).

This chapter outlines the basic costs and economic benefit inherent in the utilization of a PA in a practice, the economic framework for a medical practice, and financial analysis for the more common practice settings. Three different settings are considered, including the use of an emergency medicine PA, the outpatient primary care PA, and the surgical PA. Each scenario shares a number of different financial factors related to income generation and time attributed to the opportunity cost of physician supervision.

PRACTICE ECONOMICS AND FUNDAMENTALS

The American Academy of Physician Assistants (AAPA) Medical Group Management Association (MGMA) is an excellent source of information as it relates practice demographics and financial metrics that apply to the PA field and the larger context of a medical practice. The AAPA provides comprehensive information on salaries by clinical setting and geographic area. The MGMA, through its fee-based references, underscores the importance of recognizing the larger framework of the cost drivers of any medical practice before considering the introduction of a PA into a practice. First, a solvent practice must have the working capital or cash flow to fund the day-to-day operations and overhead of the office and staff. Services delivered today often do not receive reimbursement for 90 to 100 days. Further, the charge billed is commonly not the ultimate collection amount. Based on the experience of the authors, discount or disallowance to charges can be as high as 80% for Medicaid; they average 40% to 80% for other insurance plans.

Experts have estimated the productivity of the PA as 38% to 100% of a physician in various clinical settings.[5-7] In certain clinical practices, however, a PA can approach the productivity of a physician, minus the opportunity cost of physician supervision.[8] Billing for PA-provided services varies based upon the employment status and the requirements of contracts in effect with the physician or medical group practice (MGMA). Practice size can also influence the utilization of a PA. Experts with MGMA suggest that a medium-to-large practice can benefit most from the use of the PA.[9,10]

The Primary Care Physician Assistant

Most primary care PAs are employees—often employed by the physician, the group practice, or health/university system. A fully employed PA, in this example, sees 4500 patients per year, with an average gross charge of $125 per patient. This generates $562,500 in gross revenue before the charges to revenue. The assumption in the example as it relates to the patient's insurance status is a mix of private pay, private insurance, Medicare, and Medicaid (**Table 5-1**).

Table 5-1 Financial Analysis for Primary Care Physician Assistant

Income/Revenue (Gross)		% Tot Rev	
Office Visits	$562,500		Note 1
Procedures			Note 2
Total Revenue	$562,500		
Less:			
Receivables Carrying Cost	$5625	1%	Note 3
Billing Costs	45,000	8%	Note 4
Disallowance	196,875	35%	Note 5
Bad Debt	5625	1%	Note 6
Total Charge to Revenue	$253,125	45%	
Revenue Net of Charges	$309,375	55%	
Costs			
Salary	$80,000	14%	Note 7
Benefits	17,600	3%	Note 8
Licenses/CME	2000	0%	Note 9
Professional Liability Insurance	4800	1%	Note 10
Physician Supervision	30,938	6%	Note 11
Contribution to Overhead	123,750	22%	Note 12
Total Costs	$259,088	46%	
Net Contribution to Practice	$50,288	9%	

Note 1: 4500 visits per year with an average gross charge of $100 (MGMA)

Note 2: Included in office visit charge

Note 3: Assumes an interest rate of 4% for 90 days of gross charges

Note 4: Assumes an 8% cost of gross charges to cover the cost of all billing, collection, & cash application (MGMA)

Note 5: Assumes average charge-off of 35% for discounts and write-offs from insurance companies, Medicare, & Medicaid (MGMA)

Note 6: Assumes 1% gross charges

Note 7: Salary of PA as a general average (adapted from AAPA census)

Note 8: Assumes typical benefit package of health insurance, 401k, disability insurance, & payroll taxes (MGMA)

Note 9: Costs for medical malpractice and contribution towards licenses or related fees (AAPA insurance program)

Note 10: Assumes PA only portion of malpractice with tail through typical insurance plan and limits

Note 11: Considers a 10% lost opportunity of the supervising physician to see patients to net revenue (adapted from literature)

Note 12: Assumes a 40% of net revenue to pay for office, support staff, and supplies

The charges to gross revenue are significant: $253,125. The smaller of the charges to the gross revenue include the carrying cost of the receivable ($5625) that accounts for the time waiting to be paid by the insurance plan and the bad debt ($5625) for self-pay patients who do not pay their bill. The larger reductions to revenue are related to the billing cost ($45,000) and disallowances or discounts ($196,875) taken by the insurance plans per contractual terms with the provider or organization. The MGMA reports that billing costs are commonly around 8% of gross charges. Disallowances vary by plan and contract; the average used in this example is 35%.

For illustration purposes, the salary of the primary care PA is $80,000 annually, before other benefit or employment-related costs. In general, the primary care PA is paid close to the average salary reported by the AAPA.[11] Other employment-related costs of $17,600 assume a common benefit package of health insurance, dental insurance, 401K, disability/workmen's compensation insurance, and payroll taxes. The reimbursement for the license costs and continuing medical education (CME units) are estimated in total at $2000 annually.

The remaining two major line-item expenses include the cost of supervision and a contribution to overhead. Supervision is required for the PA in every clinical setting. The degree of supervision varies based upon the setting and the experience of the PA. An estimate adapted from the productivity differences published by the MGMA of 10% has been applied to this example, resulting in an annual expense of $30,938. Overhead is an important consideration; it includes the cost of the office, support staff, and other expenses required to run the practice. The percentage used in this example is modest at 40% of charges, totaling $123,750.

Assuming that all of the revenue and line-item cost targets are met, the PA in this example contributes $50,288 to the practice per year. As simple as this looks on paper, many factors can affect this number. Billing and collections must occur effectively and must yield the net collections projected. A poorly run billing operation can easily result in uncollected charges and a subsequent financial loss. Cost management is also important. Support staff and office occupancy costs can easily erode the financial benefit of the PA in a practice. Notably, in this example the contribution of overhead by the PA and the payment or consideration of the opportunity costs of physician supervision must be considered.

The Emergency Medicine Physician Assistant

Most emergency medicine PAs are employees. The EM PA is often employed by an emergency medicine group. In this example, a fully employed EM PA sees 4000 patients per year, with a gross charge of $200 per patient. This generates $800,000 in gross revenue before the charges to revenue. The assumption in this example as it relates to the patient insurance status is a mix of private pay, private insurance, Medicare, and Medicaid. The charge of $200 is on the lower side, given the number of PAs in emergency medicine who work in the fast-track area of the emergency department. (See **Table 5-2**).

The charges to gross revenue are significant: $288,000. The smaller of the charges to the gross revenue include the carrying cost of the receivable ($8000) that accounts for the time waiting to be paid by the insurance plan and the bad debt ($40,000) of the self-pay patients who do not pay their bill. Bad debt is higher in the emergency medicine setting due to the uninsured who receive care. The larger reductions to revenue are related to the billing cost ($64,000) and disallowances or discounts ($40,000) taken by the insurance plans per contractual terms with the provider or organization and high number of uninsured. MGMA reports that billing costs are commonly around 8% of gross charges. Disallowances vary by plan and contract; the average used in this example is 50%.

For illustration purposes, the salary of the EM PA is $100,000 annually, before other benefit or employment-related costs. In general, the EM PA is paid more than the primary care PA or the median salary reported by the AAPA.[11] Other employment-related costs of $22,000 assume a common benefit package of health insurance, dental insurance, 401K, disability/workmen's compensation insurance, and payroll taxes. The reimbursement for the license costs and continuing medical education (CME units) are estimated in total at $2000 annually. Malpractice insurance is estimated at $6000 per year.

Table 5-2 Financial Analysis for Emergency Medicine Physician Assistant

Income/Revenue (Gross)		% Tot Rev	
Office Visits	$800,000		Note 1
Procedures			Note 2
Total Revenue	$800,000		
Less:			
Receivables Carrying Cost	$8000	1%	Note 3
Billing Costs	64,000	8%	Note 4
Disallowance	400,000	50%	Note 5
Bad Debt	40,000	5%	Note 6
Total Charge to Revenue	$512,000	64%	
Revenue Net of Charges	$288,000	36%	
Costs			
Salary	$100,000	13%	Note 7
Benefits	22,000	3%	Note 8
Licenses/CME	2000	0%	Note 9
Professional Liability Insurance	6000	1%	Note 10
Physician Supervision	28,800	4%	Note 11
Contribution to Overhead	57,600	7%	Note 12
Total Costs	$216,400	27%	
Net Contribution to Practice	$71,600	9%	

Note 1: 4000 visits per year with an average gross charge of $200 (MGMA)

Note 2: Included in office visit charge

Note 3: Assumes an interest rate of 4% for 90 days of gross charges

Note 4: Assumes an 8% cost of gross charges to cover the cost of all billing, collection, & cash application (MGMA)

Note 5: Assumes average charge-off of 50% for discounts and write-offs from insurance companies, Medicare, & Medicaid (MGMA)

Note 6: Assumes 1% gross charges

Note 7: Salary of PA as a general average (adapted from AAPA census)

Note 8: Assumes typical benefit package of health insurance, 401k, disability insurance, & payroll taxes (MGMA)

Note 9: Costs for medical malpractice and contribution towards licenses or related fees (AAPA insurance program)

Note 10: Assumes PA only portion of malpractice with tail through typical insurance plan and limits

Note 11: Considers a 10% lost opportunity of the supervising physician to see patients to net revenue (adapted from literature)

Note 12: Assumes a 20% of net revenue to pay for support staff and general practice management

The remaining two major line-item expenses include the cost of supervision and a contribution to overhead. Supervision is required for the PA in every clinical setting. The degree of supervision can vary based upon the setting and experience of the PA. The estimate that has been adapted from the productivity differences published by the MGMA is 10% of net revenue and is applied to this example, resulting in a charge of $28,800. Overhead is an important line item: it covers the cost of the support staff and other expenses required to run the practice. This cost is often lower in an emergency medicine practice. The percentage used in this example is modest at 20% of charges, totaling $57,600.

Assuming that all of the revenue and line-item cost targets are met, the PA in this example contributes $71,600 per year to the practice. Again, the numbers seem straightforward. The factors that could affect these numbers are limitless. Billing and collections must occur effectively and must yield the net collections projected. A poorly run billing operation can easily result in uncollected charges and a subsequent financial loss. Coding and documentation are especially important in the emergency medicine setting. Again, cost management is important. Notably, in this example the contribution of overhead by the PA and the payment or consideration of the opportunity costs of physician supervision is considered.

THE SURGICAL PA

Many surgical PAs are contractors; that is, they are self-employed. This example assumes that a self-employed surgical PA attends 1200 cases per year with a gross charge of $475 per case. This generates $570,000 in gross revenue before the charges to revenue. The assumption in the example as it relates to the patient insurance status is a mix of private pay, private insurance, Medicare, and Medicaid. The charge of $475 is an average assumed for the financial illustration. (See **Table 5-3**).

The charges to gross revenue in this example are significant: $330,600. The smaller of the charges to the gross revenue include the carrying cost of the receivables ($5700) that accounts for the time waiting to be paid by the insurance plan and the bad debt ($17,100)

Table 5–3 Financial Analysis for Surgical Physician Assistant

Income/Revenue (Gross)		% Tot Rev	
Office Visits			
Procedures	$570,000		Note 1/ 2
Total Revenue	$570,000		
Less:			
Receivables Carrying Cost	$5700	1%	Note 3
Billing Costs	45,600	8%	Note 4
Disallowance	171,000	30%	Note 5
Bad Debt	17,100	3%	Note 6
Total Charge to Revenue	$239,400	42%	
Revenue Net of Charges	$330,600	58%	
Costs			
Salary	$110,000	19%	Note 7
Benefits	24,200	4%	Note 8
Licenses/CME	2000	0%	Note 9
Professional Liability Insurance	6000	1%	Note 10
Physician Supervision	33,060	6%	Note 11
Contribution to Overhead	66,120	12%	Note 12
Total Costs	$241,380	42%	
Net Contribution to Practice	$89,220	16%	

Note 1: 1200 cases per year with an average gross charge of $475 (MGMA)

Note 2: Included in office visit charge

Note 3: Assumes an interest rate of 4% for 90 days of gross charges

Note 4: Assumes an 8% cost of gross charges to cover the cost of all billing, collection, & cash application (MGMA)

Note 5: Assumes average charge-off of 50% for discounts and write-offs from insurance companies, Medicare, & Medicaid (MGMA)

Note 6: Assumes 3% gross charges

Note 7: Salary of PA as a general average (adapted from AAPA census)

Note 8: Assumes typical benefit package of health insurance, 401k, disability insurance & payroll taxes (MGMA)

Note 9: Costs for medical malpractice and contribution towards licenses or related fees (AAPA insurance program)

Note 10: Assumes PA only portion of malpractice with tail through typical insurance plan and limits

Note 11: Considers a 10% lost opportunity of the supervising physician to see patients to net revenue (adapted from literature)

Note 12: Assumes a 20% of net revenue to pay for support staff and general practice management for the self-pay patients who do not pay their bill. The larger reductions to revenue are related to the billing cost ($45,600) and disallowances or discounts ($171,000) taken by the insurance plans per contractual terms with the provider or organization and the high number of uninsured patients. MGMA reports that billing costs are commonly around 8% of gross charges. Disallowances vary by plan and contract; the average used in this example is 30%.

For illustration purposes, the salary of the surgical PA is $110,000 annually before other benefit or employment related costs. In general, the surgical PA is paid more than the primary care PA or the median salary reported by the AAPA.[11] The other employment-related costs of $24,200 assume a common benefit package of health insurance, dental insurance, 401K plan, disability/workmen's compensation insurance, and payroll taxes. The reimbursement for the license costs and CME units are estimated in total at $2000 annually. Malpractice insurance is estimated at $6000 per year.

The remaining two major line-item expenses include the cost of supervision and a contribution to overhead. Supervision is required for the PA in every clinical setting. The degree of supervision can vary based upon the setting and experience of the PA. The estimate that has been adapted from the productivity differences published by the MGMA is 10% of net revenue and applied to this example, resulting in a charge of $33,060. The overhead is an important line item that must be considered. It covers the cost of the support staff and other expenses required to run the practice. This cost is often lower in an emergency medicine practice. The percentage used in this example is modest at 20% of charges, totaling $66,120 annually. The collection of overhead and supervision cost from the revenue of the PA could be viewed as a financial benefit to the physician or group as a result of having a PA in the practice.

Assuming that all of the revenue and line-item cost targets are met, the PA in this example would generate a contribution to the practice of $89,220 per year. Again the numbers seem straightforward. The factors that could affect these numbers are limitless. Billing and collections must occur effectively and must yield the net collections projected. A poorly run billing operation can easily result in uncollected charges and a subsequent financial loss. Coding and documentation are especially important in the surgical setting. Notably, in this example the contribution of overhead by the PA and the payment or consideration of the opportunity costs of physician supervision is considered.

CONCLUSION

Overall, all 3 examples clearly illustrate the financial value of a PA to a practice. Non-financial benefits of employing a PA should be considered and factored as well. Physician assistants generally contribute to increasing free time and decreasing time on call for the physician. How a PA can be beneficial is a multifaceted subject. One important consideration is the professional involvement of the supervising physician as it relates to the financial statement itself. Do you know what the PA generates? How much the practice collects? What is the amount of overhead incurred by the practice? It can be difficult to achieve a particular target or goal if these elements remain unknown. Hopefully, these sample financial statements can serve as a starting point for understanding how a PA can be contributing to a successful medical practice.

REFERENCES

1. Catlin A, Cowan C, Heffler S, Washington B. Trends: National health spending in 2005: The slowdown continues. *Health Affairs.* 2007;26(1):142.
2. Menzel P, Light DW. A conservative case for universal access to health care. *The Hastings Center Report.* 2006;36(4):36.
3. Wilson JF. Primary care delivery changes as nonphysician clinicians gain independence. *Ann Intern Med.* 2008;149(8):597–600.
4. AAPA. Blueprint for change. Available at: http://aapa.org/advocacy-and-practice-resources/federal-advocacy/pas-for-a-healthy-america/blueprints-for-change. Accessed December 2, 2009.
5. Riportella-Muller R, Libby D, Kindig D. The substitution of physician assistants and nurse practitioners for physician residents in teaching hospitals. *Health Affairs.* 1995;14(2):181.
6. Record JC, ed. *Staffing primary care in 1990: Physician replacement and cost savings.* New York: Springer; 1981.

7. Schweitzer SO, McCally M, Blomquist RJ, Berger BD, McCabe M, eds. Springer Series on Health Care and Society. February 1981; 6:115–127.

8. Cyr KA. Physician–PA practice in a military clinic: A statistical comparison of productivity/availability. *Physician Assistant.* April 1985:112–124.

9. MGMA. *Physician compensation and production survey: 2006 report based on 2005 data.* Washington, DC: Medical Group Management Assoc.; 2006.

10. Vuletich M. Crunching numbers: Medium, large practices might make better use of NPPs than small practices. *MGMA e-connexion.* 2006(97). Available at: http://www.mgma.com/pm/article.aspx?id=450. Accessed March 30, 2009.

11. Gans DN. Why nonphysician providers? *MGMA e-connexion.* 2005; 5(10):25–27. Available at: http://www3.mgma.com/articles/index.cfm?fuseaction=detail.main&articleID=13613. Accessed April 1, 2009.

12. American Academy of Physician Assistants. *2006 AAPA Physician Assistant Census Report: List of Tables and Subject Index.* Alexandria, VA: AAPA; 2006.

Chapter 6

Generational Factors

Awareness and understanding of generational cultures and attitudes are important as health professionals work together. This is particularly true with the physician–physician assistant (PA) team. Generational gaps among healthcare colleagues present unique relationship challenges. While professional behaviors such as reliability, respect for others, and attention to confidentiality are expected across all generations, perceptions of issues such as feedback, work ethic, flexibility, and use of technology vary considerably across generations. Although physician–PA teams are bound by a legal supervisory relationship, the style and details of supervisory relationships vary greatly based on the generation of each individual.

Four generations typically recognized as part of the current healthcare workforce:

- Traditionalists and/or veterans (born 1922–1945)[1]
- Boomers (born 1946–1964)[2]
- Gen X-ers (born 1965–1980)[3]
- Millenials and/or Generation Y-ers (born 1981–2000)[4]

Zemke et al. in *Generations at Work* describe generalized attitudes and points of view of each generation and purport that they are based on the historic and cultural experiences they share.[5] For example,

Traditionalists and/or veterans were impacted by their childhood experiences of the Great Depression and their subsequent roles during World War II. They are thought of as hardworking, cautious, and financially conservative. Their problem-solving style is to look to the past for insight and guidance. Loyalty, recognition of seniority, and discipline are key features of their work ethic. While most workers in this generation are expected to leave the workforce by 2011, that may not be true in health care.

BABY BOOMERS

Baby Boomers, known as the largest cohort in health care, typically grew up in nuclear families and were encouraged to be creative and to rewrite the rules. Boomers are known for their strong work ethic and see work as defining themselves and others. Boomers are widely associated with privilege because many grew up in a time of affluence. They were the healthiest and wealthiest generation until that time, and they were among the first to grow up genuinely expecting the world to improve with time.

Baby Boomers grew up in a time of relative affluence and saw themselves as "special." They were the last generation to grow up in nuclear families and are still sometimes surprised by the family variations they now see. Since they did not grow up with technology, they have had to learn these skills and are sometimes less than enthusiastic about these advancements.

GENERATION X

Generation X is defined by the breakdown of the nuclear family. Many of this generation grew up in divorced families or families where both parents worked. Some experts term this generation the *latch-key* generation. As a result, they place major importance on spending time with their own families and seek a work–life balance. Having experienced the *dot-com meltdown*, they see themselves as self-sufficient and rely on their peers for the kind of support that was formerly provided by a life-long career in a single corporation. Generation X-ers grew up with technology and are comfortable using it in all phases of life, including the job search and telecommuting. This generation prefers a more "flat" organization in terms of hierarchy and leadership. They also prefer less directive assignments and want to find their own solutions to problems and issues.

GENERATION Y (MILLENNIAL)

Generation Y workers have high expectations—of themselves and of their employers! Professional development is important to them, and they want leaders—or in this case, supervising physicians—who will promote that growth. They prefer frequent feedback and rapidly increasing responsibility. Work–life balance is also important to them, but they have high expectations of themselves, including early achievements, scheduled lives, and rewards and recognition for their hard work. They can make valuable contributions to the team as "technology experts."

The work ethic varies across the 4 generations. Veterans are loyal, disciplined, and have most likely worked with only one or two employers across their career. Boomers value a democratic work setting and often define themselves by their career. The Gen X-er work ethic is driven by their goal of work–life balance, their expectation of having multiple jobs across time, and their reliance on peers—rather than corporate structures—for support. Generation Y-ers see work as an opportunity and expect to work hard to gain new opportunities quickly.

Table 6-1 considers possible interactions between supervising physicians and PAs from the 4 generational groups and details the team's possible perceptions of issues and offers solutions.

Both formal evaluation and less formal feedback are important in building the relationship between the physician and the PA. Physicians in the "veteran" generation may be most comfortable with regular and required performance evaluations but may be less enthusiastic about feedback. Their view is often, "we'll work it out as we work together." Boomers—in their preferred "democratic" work setting, are more likely to feel that it's really "all about the relationship." Formal evaluations

Table 6–1 Work Ethic

MD Veteran/ Veteran PA	Loyal/ Disciplined	Loyal/ Disciplined	Everyone works hard	No action needed.
MD Veteran/ Boomer PA	Loyal/ Disciplined	Work Defines Me	Hard-working teams	No action needed.
MD Veteran/ X PA	Loyal/ Disciplined	Work/Life Balance	A "career" or a "job"	Clarify/ negotiate.
MD Veteran/ Mill PA	Loyal/ Disciplined	Work as Opportunity	Status quo vs. growing edges	Clarify/ assign.
MD Boomer/ Veteran PA	Work Defines Me	Loyal/ Disciplined	Team Practice	No action needed.
MD Boomer/ Boomer PA	Work Defines Me	Work Defines Me	Democratic environment	No action needed.
MD Boomer/ X PA	Work Defines Me	Work/Life Balance	"Career" vs "Job"	Clarify/ negotiate.
MD Boomer/ Mill PA	Work Defines Me	Work as Opportunity	High expectations for inclusion	Clarify/ negotiate.
MD X/Vet PA	Work/Life Balance	Loyal/ Disciplined	Potential for value disagreements	Recognize strengths.
MD X/ Boomer PA	Work/Life Balance	Work Defines Me	Potential for value disagreements	Emphasize common goals.
MD X/X PA	Work/Life Balance	Work Life Balance	Understanding/ supportive	No action needed.
MD X/ Mill PA	Work/Life Balance	Work as Opportunity	Differing expectations	Clarify/ assign.
MD Mill/ Vet PA	Work as Opportunity	Loyal/ Disciplined	Widely different work-styles	Recognize differences.
MD Mill/ Boomer PA	Work as Opportunity	Work Defines Me	Open-ended vs clearly defined	Recognize differences.
MD Mill/ X PA	Work as Opportunity	Work/Life Balance	Widely differing expectations	Clarify/ Negotiate.
MD Mill/ Mill PA	Work as Opportunity	Work as Opportunity	Expectations not clear to others	Inclusion of other workers.

and structured feedback are less important to them. Generation X-ers value feedback—and often think that it needs to go both ways—back and forth between the supervisor and the employee. This can create tension if it is not well communicated or understood. Generation Y-ers want frequent—and instant—feedback. While Generation Y-ers see this as critical to their growth and achievement, others can see this as disruptive to the team. **Table 6-2** reviews perceptions of feedback by the supervising physician, the PA, and team.

Flexibility in job expectations and scheduling can be a source of disagreement across the generations. Veterans like structure, discipline, and consistency. They may feel that flexibility is destructive to the work environment. Boomers also like structure, but they feel it

Table 6–2 Feedback/Evaluation

MD/PA	MD	PA	Team Impression	Solution
MD Veteran/ Veteran PA	Annual/ Regular Evals	Annual/ Regular Evals	Formal evals are routine	No Changes
MD Veteran/ Boomer PA	Annual/ Regular Evals	Feedback Not Valued	Evals create tension	Adhere to Schedule
MD Veteran/ X PA	Annual/ Regular Evals	Feedback Valued	Differing expectations	Compromise
MD Veteran/ Mill PA	Annual/ Regular Evals	Feedback NOW	Widely differing expectations	Acknowledge Differences
MD Boomer/ Veteran PA	Feedback Not Valued	Annual/ Regular Evals	Evals don't get done	Adhere to Schedule
MD Boomer/ Boomer PA	Feedback Not Valued	Feedback Not Valued	"What Evals?"	Compliance Strategies
MD Boomer/ X PA	Feedback Not Valued	Feedback Valued	PA asks for more	Acknowledge Differences
MD Boomer/ Mill PA	Feedback Not Valued	Feedback Now	PA demands	Review Feedback Expectations

(continues)

Table 6–2 Feedback/Evaluation (*Continued*)

MD/PA	MD	PA	Team Impression	Solution
MD X/Vet PA	Feedback Valued	Annual/ Regular Evals	Differing styles/expec- tations	Compromise
MD X/ Boomer PA	Feedback Valued	Feedback Not Valued	Issue creates tension	Acknowledge differences
MD X/X PA	Feedback Valued	Feedback Valued	Parallel expectations	No action needed
MD X/ Mill PA	Feedback Valued	Feedback Now	Lots of feedback	Acknowledge each view
MD Mill/ Vet PA	Feedback Now	Annual/ Regular Evals	REALLY dif- ferent styles/ expects	Acknowledge differences
MD Mill/ Boomer PA	Feedback Now	Feedback Not Valued	Tension over this issue	Acknowledge differences Ask for help
MD Mill/ X PA	Feedback Now	Feedback Valued	Seldom a problem	No action needed
MD Mill/ Mill PA	Feedback Now	Feedback Now	Too much feedback?	Acknowledge other team- member views

should be possible to negotiate for what they need. Generation X-ers want both flexibility and understanding with respect to their need to be with their families and to pursue their own interests. Generation Y-ers may make assumptions about flexibility that is not really there and then be unhappy with restrictions. **Table 6-3** reviews issues around flexibility.

Technology can still become a flash point in the clinical workplace. Some members of the veteran's generation would still like it to "go away," but most see it as a "necessary evil." Boomers see it as a useful tool—but also sometimes an interruption. Generation X-ers grew up with technology and are adept in its use. Generation Y-ers may quickly become the technology leaders in the clinic, but they also need to be inclusive and patient with others. **Table 6-4** reviews technology issues.

Table 6–3 Flexibility/Scheduling

MD/PA	MD	PA	Team Perceptions	Solutions
MD Veteran/ Veteran PA	Work Until Done	Work Until Done	Shared expectations	No action needed
MD Veteran/ Boomer PA	Work Until Done	Democratic Schedule	Plans shared	Communicate
MD Veteran/ X PA	Work Until Done	Negotiable Schedule	Conflicts over control	Overcommunicate
MD Veteran/ Mill PA	Work Until Done	Hard Work = Freedom	High expectations/too soon	Value other workers
MD Boomer/ Veteran PA	Democratic Schedule	Work Until Done	No major problem	No action needed
MD Boomer/ Boomer PA	Democratic Schedule	Democratic Schedule	Expectations aligned	No action needed
MD Boomer/ X PA	Democratic Schedule	Negotiable Schedule	Potential for conflict	Overcommunicate
MD Boomer/ Mill PA	Democratic Schedule	Hard Work = Freedom	Structure vs autonomy	Clarify/negotiate
MD X/Vet PA	Negotiable Schedule	Work Until Done	Potential for misunderstanding	Create flexibility for veteran
MD X/ Boomer PA	Negotiable Schedule	Democratic Schedule	Potential for misunderstanding	Overcommunicate
MD X/X PA	Negotiable Schedule	Negotiable Schedule	Expectations aligned	No action needed
MD X/ Mill PA	Negotiable Schedule	Hard Work = Freedom	Where's the structure?	Inform others Overcommunicate
MD Mill/ Vet PA	Hard Work = Freedom	Work Until Done	Confusion about getting work done	Clarify views and differing expectations
MD Mill/ Boomer PA	Hard Work = Freedom	Democratic Schedule	Conflicts in expectations	Communicate/plan
MD Mill/ X PA	Hard Work = Freedom	Negotiable Schedule	"Will anyone be here?	Reassurance
MD Mill/ Mill PA	Hard Work = Freedom	Hard Work = Freedom	Others may not understand/accept	Overcommunicate

Table 6–4 Technology

MD/PA	MD	PA	Team Perceptions	Solutions
MD Veteran/ Veteran PA	Not Me	Not Me	Don't bring it up	Outside help to avoid falling behind
MD Veteran/ Boomer PA	Not Me	Enough to Get By	Do we need this?	Accept technology need even if not valued
MDVeteran/ X PA	Not Me	I Know How	Conflicting goals	Translation/ patience/ delegation
MD Veteran/ Mill PA	Not Me	Let Me Show You	Class of cultures	Delegation/ translation
MD Boomer/ Veteran PA	Enough to Get By	Not Me	Seems impossible!	Create training and support
MD Boomer/ Boomer PA	Enough to Get By	Enough To Get By	Reluctant but resigned	Utilize younger workers/ consultants
MD Boomer/ X PA	Enough to Get By	I Can Do It	Seems doable, learn	Learn together
MD Boomer/ Mill PA	Enough to Get By	Let Me Show You	We'll do it!	Delegate, appoint young leader
MD X/Vet PA	I Can Do It	Not Me	This will take work!	Training/support
MD X/ Boomer PA	I Can Do It	Enough to Get By	A challenge	Training/clear messages
MD X/X PA	I Can Do It	I Can Do It	Shared goals	Team approach with multiple inputs
MD X/Mill PA	I Can Do It	Let Me Show You	Hang on! It's intense!	Clear communication to others

Table 6–4 Technology (*Continued*)

MD/PA	MD	PA	Team Perceptions	Solutions
MD Mill/ Vet PA	Let Me Show You	Not Me	Conflict/ stress	Basic training, celebrate accomplishments
MD Mill/ Boomer PA	Let Me Show You	Enough to Get By	How much? How fast?	Training/clear messages
MD Mill/X PA	Let Me Show You	I Can Do It	Clarifiy priorities	Inclusion/ translation
MD Mill/ Mill PA	Let Me Show You	Let Me Show You	Slow down/ include us	Include all team members

The case studies below provide examples of clinical situations where a knowledge and understanding of generational attitudes and perceptions may help both the physician and the PA in building their relationship and working together successfully. For each of these cases, consider the generational issues that impact supervision and recommend strategies for addressing these concerns based on Tables 6-1 through 6-4.

Case Study #1

Dr. Allen is a new graduate of a family medicine residency and has been hired by a community health center. She is an idealistic young woman in her late 20s who has always planned to work in a rural, underserved setting. Although she has been trained in a busy family medicine residency, she has never worked with a PA before. As one of her new responsibilities, she has been told that she will be supervising John Hubbard, a senior PA who has been with the clinic for 25 years. He is in his mid-50s and has a strong following of patients who have seen him over the years while "those young docs" have come and gone.

Case Study #2

Dr. Hill is a 68-year-old physician who has "always had a PA." In his busy internal medicine practice he has typically employed a female PA to do "that women's stuff," including gynecology and behavioral medicine. His last PA, Alexa has just retired after working with him for 15 years, and he has now hired Diana, who has been out of school for about 5 years. At 35 this is her second job.

Case Study #3

The 5-person ER Group in a medium-sized town (population 125,000) has recently chosen to hire 3 new PA graduates after having had PA students, but not PA employees, for 10 years. They are proud to have recruited 3 new graduates (all in their mid- to late 20s) who all had experience as paramedics before entering PA training. The physicians, who joined up with each other right after their residencies, are all in their 50s.

CONCLUSION

Facilitating growth and development in the presence of a generationally diverse workforce is a difficult task. Sherman, in her discussion of multigenerational nursing, makes excellent recommendations for nursing leaders who want to "enable the workforce to thrive and to meet tomorrow's health care challenges."[6] Those recommendations, listed here, should also be noted by PAs and their supervising physicians:

- Seek to understand each generational cohort and accommodate generational differences in attitudes, values, and behaviors.
- Develop generationally sensitive styles to effectively coach and motivate all members of the healthcare team.
- Develop the ability to flex a communication style to accommodate generational differences.
- Promote the resolution of generational conflict so as to build effective work teams.
- Capitalize on generational differences, using the differences to enhance the work of the entire team.[6]

REFERENCES

1. The Traditional Generation. Available at: http://www.valueoptions .com/spotlight_YIW/traditional.htm. Accessed November 29, 2010. http://www.generationsatwork.com/articles/millenials.html
2. The Baby Boomers. Available at: http://www.valueoptions.com/ spotlight_YIW/baby_boomers.htm. Accessed November 29, 2010.
3. Generation X. Available at: http://www.valueoptions.com/spotlight_ YIW/gen_x.htm. Accessed November 29, 2010.
4. Generation Y. Available at: http://www.valueoptions.com/spotlight_ YIW/gen_y.htm. Accessed November 29, 2010.
5. Zemke R, Raines C, Filipczak B. *Generations at work: Managing the clash of veterans, boomers, Xers and Nexters in your workplace.* New York, NY: AMA Publications; 2000.
6. Sherman R. Leading a multigenerational nursing workforce: issues, challenges and strategies. *Online J Iss Nursing.* 2006;11(2):manuscript 2.

Additional Readings

Lancaster LC, Stillman D. *When Generations Collide Who They Are Why They Clash, How to Solve the Generational Puzzle at Work.* New York, NY: HarperCollins; 2005.

Martin CA, Tulgan B. *Managing the Generation Mix: From Urgency to Opportunity,* Amherst, MA: HRD Press; 2006.

Precepting Physician Assistant Students

Chapter 7

An Introduction to Physician Assistant Education

When physician assistant (PA) programs were developed in the late 1960s and early 1970s, the main agenda of the federal government (which provided significant funding for the new profession) was the expansion of healthcare access with cost-effective primary care providers. However, innovative medical educators also saw PA programs as laboratories for new educational methodologies. The small size of PA classes—compared to large medical school cohorts—meant that it was relatively easy and inexpensive to try new curriculum designs. With less cost, it was also possible to discard ideas that were not successful.[1]

In addition, the regional distribution of the first PA programs created a culture for PA education that allowed PA programs to "bloom where they were planted," meaning that a wide range of curriculum designs were often accepted, depending on either the host institution (e.g., medical schools, hospitals, community colleges, or liberal arts colleges) or the healthcare delivery system in a specific region (e.g., in areas with large teaching hospitals as compared to more rural areas with extensive primary care systems). Even after 40 years, the accreditation requirements of the accrediting body for

PA programs—the Accreditation Review Commission for the Physician Assistant Education (ARC-PA)—are broad rather than specific in nature, allowing PA education to be offered in a wide range of settings and institutions. (A Web link to the ARC-PA standards is included in Appendix A).

From the beginning, the accreditation process for PA educational programs has included input from a variety of stakeholders who actively participate in the process by serving as members of the ARC-PA. These stakeholders include the following:

- The American Academy of Family Physicians
- The American Academy of Pediatrics
- The American Academy of Physician Assistants
- The American College of Physicians
- The American College of Surgeons
- The American Medical Association
- The Physician Assistant Education Association

Overall the principle question that arose—as PA educational programs were designed and implemented—was this: "How is it possible to get everything PAs need to know into the typical 2-year PA program—when it takes so much longer to educate physicians?" Several answers to this question were given:

1. It was important to be clear that *PA programs were not training physicians—or physician substitutes.* This was clearly demonstrated by the legal requirement for physician supervision as the basis for PA practice.

2. *PA programs were required to train generalists* rather than emphasize specialty practice. A key feature of the PA profession is this generalist foundation, which allows PAs to be "customized" in a specific practice setting where the supervising physician legally determines the individual scope of practice and creates opportunities for the individual PA to gain and develop skill sets specific to the clinical setting. With this model, PAs can flexibly respond to the changing healthcare system by moving

among the physician "specialties" based on individual interest or job availability.

3. *The certification process for PAs* (administered by the National Commission on Certification of Physician Assistants) *is designed to reinforce the generalist concept.* The *entry-level exam* (required by all states for PA licensure) is a generalist exam as is the *recertification exam* that is required every 6 years.

4. While all PA programs include some basic science content, courses such as anatomy and physiology are required prerequisites. This is not the case with medical school admissions. Overall, *the emphasis is on focused generalist content*, frequent testing and feedback, structured and integrated didactic course content with well-defined objectives, and clinical rotations designed to give a broad exposure to the healthcare system.

The *Standards* acknowledge the ongoing evolution of the PA profession and continue to endorse competency-based education as a fundamental tenet of PA education. They reflect the best wisdom of PA educators, accreditors, and administrators.

COMPETENCY-BASED TRAINING

Competency-based training has been a defining feature of PA education. The ARC-PA standards establish this by saying, "The *Standards* acknowledge the ongoing evolution of the PA profession and continue to endorse competency-based education as a fundamental tenet of PA education."[2]

Particularly adaptable to the needs of adult learners, competency-based training determines the outcomes or "competencies" that are expected for graduates as the first step in the creation of coursework. Competencies may be content-oriented (e.g., knowledge, skills, and attitudes) or quantitative (e.g., students must achieve a score of 80% in order to move on in the program.) Working backward from those competencies, faculty members create specific objectives—with matching assessment tools—to give clear messages to students about what is to be learned. For the PA field, the creation of the new career involved deciding what functions they would perform and then developing integrated coursework to efficiently deliver the curriculum. Competency-based training emphasizes collaboration—rather than competition—between students, thus reinforcing the ability of PAs to effectively function in teams.

CLINICAL EXPERIENCE AND/OR DEGREES

While the first PAs were military corpsmen and medics with extensive clinical experience, others with training and experience in nursing and allied health soon joined them. Most of the first programs required clinical experience, although others chose students with a more academic point of view. Although a wide range of "prerequisites" (clinical experience and academic coursework) continues, the PA career has become more degree oriented over the past 40 years. Currently, most programs offer master's degrees, although bachelor's degrees and certificates are still available. In the newly approved accreditation standards, ARC-PA is recommending that master's degrees be fully implemented in all PA programs by 2021.

The nurse practitioner (NP) field, due to its goal of achieving independent practice, plans to transition all NP programs to Doctorate in Nursing Practice programs by 2015. In comparison, PAs, with the emphasis on their relationship with supervising physicians, have not chosen to make this move.

Overall, the concern has been that increased academic degrees increase the cost of education and create barriers for the individuals who have traditionally chosen PA training, including military corpsmen, rural residents with less access to higher education, and candidates from educationally disadvantaged backgrounds.

ADMINISTRATIVE STRUCTURE

The sponsoring institution is required to provide appropriate resources for the program, including classrooms and office space, access to university services for students, and funds for appropriate levels of staffing.

All PA programs are required to have a full-time program director—a PA or a physician as well as a medical director (MD or DO) who reports to the program director. While the ARC-PA does not recommend specific faculty:student ratios, a typical program employs multiple PA faculty members who have responsibilities in both the didactic and clinical phases of the program. In addition to these faculty members, more senior faculty members serve as didactic coordinators and clinical coordinators. Individual courses are chaired by PA faculty members who are responsible for course content, delivery, curricula, and student assessment.

According to the ARC-PA Standard A2.05, core program faculty must have responsibility for the following:

1. Developing the mission statement for the program
2. Selecting applicants for admission to the PA program
3. Providing student instruction
4. Evaluating PA student performance
5. Academic counseling of PA students
6. Assuring the availability of remedial instruction
7. Designing, implementing, coordinating, and evaluating curriculum
8. Administering and evaluating the program

PA programs also employ staff members to support the faculty in managing administrative functions as well as the didactic and clinical components. The number of staff members varies widely depending upon the number of students enrolled as well as upon the complexity of the program's curriculum and the geographic distribution of the program's clinical training sites.

ADMISSIONS

Just as PA programs created the opportunity for medical educators to experiment with new curriculum designs, new admissions processes were also developed.

Acknowledging that the PA profession was attracting unique candidates (e.g., military corpsmen and medics) and that the PA role might demand new attitudes, some new PA program leaders moved away from the traditional "high-stakes" medical school interview model to processes that emphasize teamwork and problem solving.

Anecdotally, several programs adopted a full day, group interview process developed by the Peace Corps. Interviewers often included stakeholders for the new career including physicians, administrators, and consumers.

Presently, the admissions process for most PA programs—and PA candidates—begins with an electronic application process—similar to the AMCAS process for medical students called the Central Application Service for Physician Assistants (CASPA). It is rare for PA programs NOT to interview their candidates—although the interview process varies widely.

DIDACTIC EDUCATION

The broad ARC-PA Standards[2] lists requires content but does not detail requirements for total hours or course titles.

Basic science requirements include the following:

- Anatomy
- Physiology
- Pathophysiology
- Pharmacology and pharmacotherapeutics
- Genetic and molecular mechanisms of health and disease[2]

Data collection, documentation, and communication have been emphasized from the first days of PA education. These requirements are based on the understanding that supervising physicians—and other members of the healthcare team—need to have absolute confidence in consistent, compulsive, and clearly communicated history-taking and physical examination. The requirements include "instruction in interpersonal and communication skills that result in the effective exchange of information and collaboration with patients, their families, and other health professionals."[3]

Patient assessment and management requirements include the following:

1. Techniques of interviewing and eliciting a medical history
2. Performance of physical examinations across the life span
3. Generation of differential diagnoses
4. Ordering and interpretation of diagnostic studies
5. Development and implementation of treatment plans
6. Presentation of patient data in oral form
7. Documentation of patient data
8. Appropriate referral of patients[3]

MEDICINE AND PATIENT CARE

The *Standards* required that program instruction include clinical medicine covering all organ systems (standard B3.03[2]) as well as in technical skills and procedures based on current professional practice (standard B.3.05[3]).

The *Standards* specify instruction in the following aspects of patient care (standard B3.04[2]):

- Preventive
- Acute
- Chronic
- Rehabilitative
- End-of-life

BEHAVIORAL AND SOCIAL SCIENCES

PAs are expected to have strong behavioral medicine skills. Counseling and patient education skills are delineated in standard B4.01[2] and include the ability to assist patients and families in coping with illness and injury, adhering to prescribed treatment plans, and modifying their behaviors to more healthful patterns.

Standard B4.02[2] requires programs to provide instruction in normal psychological development of pediatric, adult, and geriatric patients, the detection and treatment of substance abuse; human sexuality; end-of-life issues; response to illness, injury, and stress; and principles of violence identification and prevention.

INFORMATION LITERACY

Information literacy is a relatively new requirement designed

> to equip students with the necessary skills to search, interpret, and evaluate the medical literature in order to maintain a critical, current, and operational knowledge of new medical findings including its application to individualized patient care. (Standard B5.01[2])

HEALTH POLICY

PA students are required to be knowledgeable about health policy issues (standard B6.01[2]) including the following:

1. The impact of socioeconomic issues affecting health care
2. Healthcare delivery systems and health policy
3. Reimbursement, including documentation, coding, and billing
4. Quality assurance and risk management in medical practice
5. Legal issues of health care
6. Cultural issues and their impact on healthcare policy

ETHICS

Medical ethics content (standard B6.02[2]) must include instruction in the attributes of respect for self and others, professional responsibility, the concepts of privilege, confidentiality, and informed patient consent and a commitment to the patient's welfare.

PHYSICIAN ASSISTANT PROFESSIONAL ISSUES

Physician assistant issues are typically covered in a PA role course; however, this content can also be integrated into other program courses. Standard B6.03[2] requires course content on the following topics:

1. The history of the PA profession
2. Current trends of the PA profession
3. The physician–PA team relationship
4. Political and legal issues that affect PA practice
5. PA professional organizations
6. PA program accreditation
7. PA certification and recertification
8. Licensure
9. Credentialing
10. Professional liability
11. Laws and regulations regarding prescriptive practice

CLINICAL ROTATIONS

While clinical rotations make up over half of the total PA educational experience, this is still considered a relatively short period of time. As a result, PA programs provide greater oversight over PA clinical students than would be typically seen in longer physician programs. Attendance is required, and students return to the program regularly for additional content and assessments. In addition, programs conduct site visits on students, require that students maintain electronic logs of patient encounters, and include research and community service projects in the assignments for the year.

The *Standards* require that students be provided with clinical experiences in outpatient and inpatient settings, emergency rooms or departments, long-term care, and the operating room. (B7.04) The

Standards also say that "clinical practice experiences should occur with residency trained physicians or other licensed health care professionals experienced in the following disciplines: emergency medicine, family medicine, general internal medicine, general surgery, general pediatrics, psychiatry and obstetrics/gynecology."[4]

The *Standards*[2] are more explicit in standard B7.03 about specific types of care by requiring that programs

document patient experiences with patients seeking the following:

a) Medical care across the life span to include, infants, children, adolescents, adults, and the elderly
b) Prenatal care and women's health care
c) Care for conditions requiring inpatient surgical management, including preoperative, intraoperative, and postoperative care
d) Care for conditions requiring emergency management
e) Care for psychiatric/behavioral conditions

The issue of international rotations is a growing opportunity for PA educational programs. The 4th edition of the *Standards*[5] contains more specific requirements for these types of experiences to assure formal approval, structured monitoring of students, and the provision of appropriate "safety nets" during these rotations.

NEW CONTENT

Because it is easier to make changes in PA curriculum compared to the complex medical school process, PA programs regularly and frequently update and add content. Often these decisions are made to make graduates more marketable in the rapidly changing marketplace. For example, typical new additions to PA didactic curriculum have included informatics (including exposure to electronic medical records), evidence-based medicine, genetics, palliative care, the prevention of medical errors, and new delivery system models such as the medical home. Many supervising preceptors look forward to hearing about this new content from their students!

LICENSING AND CREDENTIALING

Graduates of ARC-PA accredited programs are eligible to take the entry-level exam offered by the National Commission on Certification of Physician Assistants. This exam is required for licensure—which occurs at the state level.

REFERENCES

1. Morton-Rias D, Hammond J. Education. In: Ballweg R, Sullivan E, Brown D, Vetrosky D, eds. *Physician Assistant: A Guide to Clinical Practice.* Philadelphia, PA: Saunders Elsevier; 2007:44–60.
2. ARC-PA. Accreditation Standards for Physician Assistant Education. 3rd ed. September 1, 2006. Available at: http://www.arc-pa.org/documents/3rdeditionwithPDchangesandregionals4.24.08a.pdf. Accessed February 13, 2011.
3. ARC-PA. Accreditation Standards for Physician Assistant Education. 3rd ed. September 1, 2006: 12. Available at: http://www.arc-pa.org/documents/StdsandCompetencies3.24.06.pdf. Accessed February 13, 2011.
4. ARC-PA. Accreditation Standards for Physician Assistant Education. 3rd ed. September 1, 2006: 14. Available at: http://www.arc-pa.org/documents/StdsandCompetencies3.24.06.pdf. Accessed February 13, 2011.
5. ARC-PA. Accreditation Standards for Physician Assistant Education, 4th ed. Effective September 1, 2010. Available at: http://www.arc-pa.org/documents/Standards4theditionFINALwithclarifyingchangesJuly2010.pdf. Accessed February 13, 2011.

Chapter 8

The Clinical Experience

Healthcare providers welcome physician assistant (PA) students into their practices for a number of reasons. Some teach to give back to their profession; others enjoy the intellectual atmosphere created when a student challenges them with a question. Regardless of the reason, this chapter provides valuable insight into some aspects of student–preceptor relationship and PA education in clinical practice, such as the preceptor characteristics that students prefer, whether a PA student slows down the office practice, tailoring the clinical experience to be more learning centered, and the tools that can be used for effective and efficient teaching.

Physician assistants are licensed to practice medicine and to deliver patient care in all medical and surgical specialties with physician supervision.[1] To obtain state licensure, PAs must pass a national certifying examination administered by the National Commission on Certification of Physician Assistants (NCCPA). Eligibility for the examination is granted upon graduation from an accredited training program. The educational training of PAs is typically delivered through a curricular model that includes classroom and laboratory instruction followed by clinical rotations. The series of clinical rotations that PA students complete is commonly referred to as the "clerkship experience." After a brief discussion of the antecedents to and the logistics of clinical rotations, this chapter presents methods to enhance the clerkship experience for both the PA student and the preceptor.

In the United States in 2008, more that 73,800 PAs were in clinical practice; they were graduates of more than 140 accredited PA training programs.[1] The average PA program is 26 months in duration and consists of more than 3200 contact hours of instruction.[1-3] Regardless of the mission or location of the sponsoring institution, the instructional model for PA education is based on two central themes: a practice that is physician-dependent and an education that is competency based.[2] Beginning with Duke University (sponsor of the first PA program) in 1965 and continuing today, the curriculum blueprint used by most PA programs resembles that of medical schools. It consists of two training stages: the preclinical (didactic) phase and the clinical rotations (clerkship experience).[2,4] The didactic segment is designed to provide each student with the knowledge, skills, and attitudes (KSAs) necessary to advance from the classroom to clinical rotations. The intention of the clerkship phase of training is to allow the PA students to combine classroom learning with actual patient care; to expand their understanding of patient assessment and disease management; and to develop the competencies required to graduate, pass the NCCPA certifying examination, and enter practice. This stage of training creates an environment of individualized, learner-focused training and provides a mentoring opportunity for the preceptor. Each program and its faculty are responsible for developing learning objectives that describe the educational goals that should be completed during all courses and clinical rotations. These objectives serve as a roadmap to guide student and preceptor efforts and to promote mastery.

Physician assistant students complete more than 1150 hours of classroom and laboratory instruction (more than 400 hours in the basic sciences, 175 hours in the behavioral sciences, and nearly 580 hours in clinical medicine) prior to their clinical rotations.[1,5] The clerkship experience consists of 2000 hours (an average of 51.5 weeks) of patient contact under the supervision and direction of a preceptor, most commonly a physician (DO or MD), PA, or nurse practitioner (NP).[1-3] Students gain experience in both inpatient and outpatient facilities, completing a series of rotations that range in length from 2 to 10 weeks.[4] The clerkship experience includes both required and elective rotations. The PA student participates in the diagnosis and management of a diverse mix of patients during rotations that include emergency medicine, family medicine, internal medicine, general surgery, geriatrics, pediatrics, and obstetrics/gynecology.[2-5] Students' clinical skills are refined and expanded as they progress through the clerkship phase of their training. The diverse nature of the rotations ensures broad-based exposure to patient problems that prepare the PA student for practice as a primary-care provider or in a medical or surgical specialty. The teaching and feedback offered by preceptors, the completion of assigned reading and learning activities, and summative end-of-rotation assessments, work together to assure a well-rounded educational experience for the PA student.

The clerkship experience for students usually occurs in a randomly sequenced manner. Although programs create learning objectives for each rotation, it is not unusual for students—even those working with the same preceptor—to describe the experience as unstructured and haphazard.[6] This can happen for a number of reasons. Students enter the clerkship experience with differing expectations, degrees of ability, and levels of motivation. Preceptors possess varying levels of teaching ability. The degree of supervision and quality of teaching provided by preceptors may not be consistent across sites. There are seasonal and economic variables that alter the nature of certain medical specialties. For example, a rotation in pediatrics during the winter (i.e., primarily respiratory illnesses) differs greatly from a rotation at the same facility in July (i.e., more sports-related injuries). The effectiveness of the PA student's clerkship experience is therefore determined by the interaction of four key variables: (1) the learning objectives established by the PA program, (2) the learning style of the PA student, (3) the teaching style of the preceptor, and (4) the clinical environment (see **Figure 8-1**). The greater the degree of interface among these variables, the more likely the result will be successful PA student learning, preceptor fulfillment, patient satisfaction, and, thereby, PA program effectiveness.

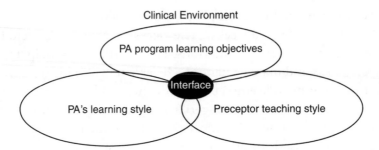

Figure 8–1 Key Variables in the Physician Assistant Student's Learning Environment.

Source: From Smith P, Morrison J. Clinical clerkships: students can structure their own learning. *Med Educ.* September 2006;40(9):884-92.

The prototypical day-in-the-office involves the following activity repeated several times: (a) PA student sees a patient, presents the history and physical examination findings, then offers a diagnosis, next steps, and a therapeutic plan (when warranted); (b) the preceptor evaluates the patient; and (c) the preceptor offers feedback to the PA student. Potential challenges that programs face from preceptors include concern about their teaching aptitude, the time commitment required to teach, the probable loss of clinical productivity (i.e., ability to see fewer patients), the impact that student teaching might have on patient satisfaction, and possible learner–preceptor conflicts associated with student teaching activities.[7] A number of teaching tools and faculty development opportunities exist to enhance the learning environment and reduce preceptor concerns. An appreciation of learner differences, the use of learning contracts, effective time-management and teaching strategies, knowing which teacher characteristics learners prefer, and having an understanding of how to handle the difficult student are skill sets that can improve the clerkship experience for the PA student and the preceptor.

Learning contracts have been touted as useful instruments for providing student-specific structure in the clerkship experience.[8] As defined, learning contracts are a set of learning outcomes created by the PA student that he or she expects to achieve by the end of the clerkship experience. Learning contracts are most effective when they are understood and agreed to by both the PA student and the preceptor at the beginning of the rotation. Such student-specific learning goals may include medical knowledge, procedural skills, and/or behavioral goals. On the first day of a rotation, the student and the preceptor should discuss the outcomes in the learning contract (3 to 5 outcomes are adequate) as well as details for each goal to ensure that they are explicit, measurable, and attainable.[8] An example of a very simple learning contract might include the following: by the end of the rotation, the PA student intends to be able (1) to better differentiate systolic and diastolic murmurs, (2) to identify the presence of lobar consolidation using auscultation, percussion, fremitus, and egophony, and (3) to do a patient-specific review-of-systems in less than 5 minutes.

The average time that a preceptor spends per patient visit (15.3 minutes without a student present) increases with a student present (to 16.2 minutes); this change is not statistically significant.[9] The same study reported that although the patient's time spent with the preceptor was reduced an average of 24 seconds, the patient spent an average of 12.9 minutes with the student. Whether the additional time spent with the student resulted in any change in patient satisfaction during the visit was not determined. To improve the effectiveness and efficiency of the teaching encounter the "One-Minute Preceptor" model (also known as the "Five-Step Microskills Model of Clinical Teaching") was designed. This instrument consists of 5 items that help preceptors provide students with explicit feedback (see **Table 8-1**).[10] Although originally designed as a specific sequence of items, recent literature suggests that the order of the questions and feedback statements need not be rigid.[11]

A PA student presents an example of the One-Minute Preceptor model as follows[10]:

> A 74-year-old male presents complaining of increasing shortness of breath for 2 months. He denies chest pain and orthopnea. His physical examination is positive for a diastolic murmur. I'd like to order some diagnostic studies and prescribe penicillin for endocarditis prophylaxis.

Table 8-1 The Five-Step Microskills Model of Clinical Teaching

Microskill	Example
1. Get a commitment	What is this patient's diagnosis?
2. Probe for supporting evidence	What elements of the history and/or physical examination lead you to that conclusion?
3. Teach general rules (not specific details)	Ordering an echocardiogram as follow-up will quantify the severity of the regurgitant blood flow and the nature of the valvular lesion.
4. Reinforce what was done right	The auscultatory techniques that you used to identify the diastolic murmur and its associated findings were the appropriate choices.
5. Correct mistakes	Prescribing the antibiotic that you suggested is not necessary in this situation. Please read more about this condition and the indications for prophylaxis.

Source: Parrot S, Dobbie A, Chumley H, Tysinger JW. Evidence-based office teaching—the five-step microskills model of clinical teaching. *Fam Med.* 2006;38(3):164-167. Reprinted with permission from the Society of Teachers of Family Medicine. Available at: www.stfm.org.

The student considers the following questions: (1) What is this patient's specific diagnosis? and (2) What elements of the history and/or physical examination support this conclusion? The follow-up discussion includes the following: (3) teaching general rules, (4) reinforcing what was done correctly, and (5) correcting mistakes. The focused nature of this approach is structured to motivate students to expand the patient-oriented learning experience through further reading in the medical literature. Allowing the student to see the same patients during follow-up visits reinforces the learning experience. However, the preceptor needs to avoid common mistakes associated with this teaching model: (1) taking over the case, (2) lecturing, (3) asking closed-ended questions, and (4) pushing learners beyond their readiness.[10]

Preceptors who have the teaching characteristics that students identify as most desirable can help motivate students to learn.[12] Based on the literature and anecdotal observations shared by colleagues, the most commonly cited characteristics and teaching strategies of preceptors valued most by students are these:

1. Allowing students to see patients first
2. Providing the student with increasing levels of responsibility
3. Behaving in a cheerful and enthusiastic manner
4. Asking explicit and focused questions and providing formative feedback tailored to the level of the student
5. Exposing students to procedures and allowing them to practice the skill
6. Assist the student with chart preparation (writing SOAP notes)
7. Serving as professional role models[9,12]

It is the responsibility of a preceptor to understand the individual and unique learning needs of each PA student. A perceived difficult learner situation may simply be a mismatch between the PA student's learning style and the preceptor's teaching style. When the issue of a difficult learner extends beyond this theme, however, the preceptor should contact the program for guidance. Initial communication of expectations, frequent and timely formative feedback, and candid and frequent communication with students cannot be overemphasized.

In conclusion, the clerkship experience is the responsibility of several stakeholders and can be the source of much fulfillment. The training that occurs while the PA student completes clinical rotations must be approached as a dynamic event occurring in a dynamic environment. PA programs, preceptors, and students must collaborate to create, maintain, and further develop robust environments that foster learning. The clerkship experience is a time of transformation. Creating a learning environment that provides adequate support and direction while challenging the PA student's abilities augments their development. The PA student is quickly approaching graduation and gaining the skill sets necessary to deliver effective patient care as a member of the PA–physician team. Through deliberate planning coupled with the use of evidence-based learning instruments and teaching techniques, the metamorphosis from PA student to PA is facilitated.

REFERENCES

1. American Academy of Physician Assistants Web site. PA Facts: What is a Physician Assistant? May 2009. Available at: http://www.aapa.org. Accessed October 19, 2009.
2. Jones PE. Physician assistant education in the United States. *Acad Med.* 2007;82:882–887.
3. Cawley JF. Physician assistant education: An abbreviated history. *J Physician Assist Educ.* 2007;18:6–15.
4. Association of Physician Assistant Programs. *Nineteenth Annual Report on Physician Assistant Educational Programs in the United States, 2002–2003.* Alexandria, VA: AAPA.
5. American Academy of Physician Assistants Web site. PA Facts: How to become a physician assistant. May 2009. Available at: http://www.aapa .org. Accessed October 19, 2009.
6. Smith P, Morrison J. Clinical clerkships: students can structure their own learning. *Med Educ.* 2006;40:884–892.
7. Alguire PC, DeWitt DE, Pinksy LE, Ferenchick GS. *Teaching in Your Office: A Guide to Instructing Medical Students and Residents.* Philadelphia, PA: American College of Physicians; 2001.
8. McGrae McDermott M, Curry RH, Stille FC, Martin GJ. Use of learning contracts in an office-based primary care clerkship. *Med Educ.* 1999;33:374–381.
9. Usatine RP, Tremoulet PT, Irby D. Time-efficient preceptors in ambulatory care settings. *Acad Med.* 2000;75:639–642.
10. Neher JO, Stevens N. The one-minute preceptor: Shaping the teaching conversation. *Family Med.* 2003;35:391–393.
11. Parrott S, Dobbie A, Chumley H, Tysinger JW. Evidence-based office teaching: The five-step microskills model of clinical teaching. *Fam Med.* 2006:38:164–167.
12. Fields S, Usatine R, Steiner E. Teaching medical students in the ambulatory setting. *JAMA.* 2000;283:2362–2364.

Chapter 9

Precepting Requirements, Guidelines, and Responsibilities

The act of precepting students is a tangible way physicians, PAs, and NPs can give back to their medical profession. Most clinicians recall a preceptor who taught them important medical knowledge, who pushed them to learn, and who supported them when they struggled. Excellent precepting requires the following: an environment conducive to learning, a few easily learned teaching skills, and clear expectations of what constitutes student success.

Precepting is best performed in a clinical practice environment that is conducive to teaching activities. Key requirements include two factors:

- Acknowledgement by the practice of the value of teaching
- Agreements that spell out responsibility for student oversight, patient care, and liability

Preceptors may be relieved of some of the pressures of teaching, or they may be rewarded for the extra work of teaching in a number of ways. Teaching may be part of the routine job description where everyone participates in precepting and where the practice includes teaching in compensation. This is most common in academic practice. Those not in academic settings may be able to arrange reduced productivity expectations or extra support staff when precepting. Others may have regular patient schedules while precepting, and may be rewarded for their extra time by receiving time away or financial support to attend teaching conferences, teaching rounds, or similar activities. Long-term success of precepting requires a positive benefit for the preceptor because of the added pressure of these activities during the work day.

Preceptors want to be protected from negative or unexpected medical consequences from teaching students in their daily practice. Formal agreements between the school and the preceptor covering patient care and liability are essential. Liability coverage should include indemnity for student errors, good faith oversight definitions, and specifics of the coverage. Areas in which teaching is not appropriate should be outlined clearly. These may include specific procedures or other areas of the provider's scope of practice where teaching will not occur. Billing and reimbursement issues may also limit teaching. Clear affiliation agreements between the preceptor, the practice, and the school can prevent negative outcomes from the clinical precepting arrangement.

Guidelines for precepting are best thought of as a set of techniques that allow the preceptor to teach in a structured manner in an unstructured environment. The following practice and teaching techniques can help create an optimum teaching environment:

Morning huddle. The morning huddle is a brief meeting of everyone on the healthcare team before seeing the first patient. The huddle is used by the provider and staff to plan their work day. Including the student in the huddle creates structure for the student's day by planning the patients for them to see. A brief meeting of the preceptor and student can be used to review any assignments, reporting on test results, or other follow up from patients seen the day before. The meeting can also highlight learning opportunities in the current work day.

Real-time feedback. Real-time feedback happens as students present their patients to the preceptor. During this process, the student and the preceptor use pertinent positives and negatives of the case to match "illness scripts." A more advanced student will be able to provide a more detailed presentation leading to a proposed diagnosis. These details include more thoughtful reasons that the proposed diagnosis is correct and more detailed reasons that the proposed diagnosis is not something else. It is valid to judge a student's medical knowledge based on their ability to present pertinent positives and negatives.[1] Asking questions to ensure understanding and then making a teaching point allows the preceptor to effectively and efficiently teach during patient care. The one-minute preceptor model[2] and the ask–tell–ask technique[3] describe this process in more detail.

Summative feedback. Summative evaluation should be an outcome of daily feedback. Sometimes students do not recognize that they are getting informal formative feedback and may entirely miss specific feedback in a preceptor's comparison of their progress to expectations in summative feedback. To avoid this, timely, clear, well-communicated, and specific evaluations are important.

For example a preceptor might say, "I'm going to sit down with you now and let you know what went well today, what could be better, and what you need to do to improve."

This approach may seem overly direct, but such approaches are appropriate to ensure that the student recognizes that he or she is being evaluated.

"Good job today" is much less useful than specific feedback like, "I liked the way you calmed Mr. Jones before injecting local anesthetic for the laceration repair." Using a direct approach makes evaluations of the student at the end of the rotation much easier, and such comments will not be a surprise for the student (see **Table 9-1**).

One key responsibility of a preceptor is to provide a role model for the profession; another is to be an active teacher. Being a role model means both acting and verbalizing the professional behavior expected of medical providers every day. Students benefit from hearing explanations of professional behavior and from adding to their own observations. Important behaviors to discuss are treating patients with respect, following privacy guidelines, and confronting

Table 9–1 Teaching Tips

✓ Communicate often.

✓ Use small chunks of information.

✓ Reward positive behavior – it will be repeated.

✓ Substitute "I like when you did ___" for "good job."

✓ Say "You need to improve ____" rather than nothing.

✓ Have fun, you are creating a future preceptor when you teach.

Source: From Vorvick LJ, Avnon T, Emmett RS, Robins L. Improving teaching by teaching feedback. *Med Educ.* 2008;42(5): 540-541.

unprofessional behavior in colleagues. In addition to teaching professional behavior, preceptors need to set high but reasonable expectations for student performance. After expectations are clear, teaching should be focused on clinical tools and on communicating knowledge the student needs to meet those expectations. Teaching also requires professional behavior that treats the student with respect; teaching must be free from discrimination, harassment, demoralizing, and degrading experiences.

Finally, it is important that preceptors give students honest evaluations of their medical skills and professional behavior. PA programs require a summative evaluation; some require the preceptor and student to discuss the evaluation, which is a good idea whether or not it is required. Preceptors can request help from the PA program about poor performance or difficult professionalism issues.

REFERENCES

1. Bowen JL. Educational strategies to promote clinical diagnostic reasoning. *N Engl J Med.* 2006;355(21):2217-2225.
2. Parrot S, Dobbie A, Chumley H, Tysinger JW. Evidence-based office teaching—the five-step microskills model of clinical teaching. *Fam Med.* 2006;38(3):164-167.
3. Vorvick LJ, Avnon T, Emmett RS, Robins L. Improving teaching by teaching feedback. *Med Educ.* 2008;42(5):540-541.

Chapter *Chapter* **10**

Clinical Teaching Guidelines

Clinical teaching is a crucial component of physician assistant (PA) education. This element of the educational program enables PA students to place their theoretical learning into a practical context. It is common knowedge that students become better clinicians if they learn in the context of clinical practice. Clinical teaching is also important because this education usually occurs with patients present.

Teaching in any clinical setting is difficult to plan, is highly dependent on context, and is constantly challenged by ever-changing practice demands. When used appropriately, however, these challenges can provide unique opportunities for effective teaching. Preceptors (whether it be a practicing PA or physician) are generally willing and excited for the opportunity to work with PA students and preceptors possess a desire to "give back" to the profession for the opportunities they received as students.[1] They are clinicians who have the ability to balance clinical responsibilities with student education. A good preceptor orchestrates the student rotation by doing the following:

1. Planning for the experience
2. Providing an orientation
3. Reviewing educational objectives

4. Overseeing the student's role
5. Teaching/clinically mentoring the student's activities
6. Completing student evaluations

PLANNING

The clinical preceptor usually receives notification of a student assignment from the educational program many months before the clinical rotation begins. It is appropriate for the preceptor to send a welcoming letter to the student with an invitation for a formal meeting on the first day of the rotation. Different PA programs provide different time durations for the clinical rotations. The most common rotations are between 4 and 6 weeks in length.

It is also important for the preceptor to inform the clinical staff and to make any necessary scheduling adjustments to support both orientation and supervision activities. A few days before the student arrives, the preceptor should remind the staff. The preceptor may identify scheduled patients for the student to see during the first week with the preceptor. It is not uncommon for staff to post a notice in the waiting room to inform patients that a PA student will be working in the practice. A typical notice would include the student's name, the name of the supporting academic institution, and the length of the rotation.

ORIENTATION

The orientation meeting should occur on the first day or as soon as possible after the student's arrival. This meeting sets the tone for the relationship between the student and the preceptor and typically is scheduled for at least 1 hour. A review of expectations from both the preceptor's and the student's perspectives is important, as well as a review of the clinical rotation objectives. The preceptor should introduce the student to the staff, provide a workspace for the student, and give a short tour of the clinic and/or hospital. It is also important for the preceptor to orient the student about any cultural aspects of the patient population and any unique practices and/or organizational policies. The orientation is also a good time to review daily schedule expectations, logistic details, dress code, and procedures pertaining to absences.

EDUCATIONAL OBJECTIVES

It is important for the preceptor to review any requirements of the PA program. In particular, the preceptor should review the clinical rotation objectives provided by the educational program and plan methods for the student to accomplish those objectives during their stay in the practice. In addition, the preceptor may include a set of clinical skills expected of the student.

OVERSIGHT

The preceptor must coordinate the student's educational activities during his or her clinical experience. This should include daily schedules, assigning patients to be seen, and informing patients of the student's role in the practice. "Observational" as well as "hands on" experiences may be included at different times.

TEACHING

Direct clinical teaching is the very core of the clinical experience. Effective preceptors possess a unique set of skills: proficiency in communication, ability to create a positive learning environment, and provision of constructive feedback. This experience should include self-evaluation by the student, a regular schedule of observed patient encounters, feedback from the preceptor, problem solving, and evaluation. PA students should be treated as colleagues and should be challenged to be active participants in achieving their goals and objectives.

Teaching methods and tools vary by practice, personality, and experience. Some teaching options available to the preceptor are discussed here.

Mini-Lectures

Mini-lectures are usually about 10 minutes long; they provide information or direction to the student. This method is useful as a preface or follow-up to a series of patient visits. Conversely, the student may be assigned a topic on which to prepare and then present a 10-minute lecture to the preceptor and/or staff.

Questioning

Questioning, sometimes called "pimping," involves the student in the learning process and facilitates a free flow of information and/or opinions. While closed-ended questions may be useful for data collection, open-ended questions foster better discussions between preceptor and student. This method is also useful in challenging the student to make predictions, to develop hypotheses, to defend an action, or to justify a decision.

Demonstration/Observation

Demonstration of skills by the preceptor is an integral component of the clinical experience. This includes patient interviewing skills, physical examination skills, and procedural skills. Then, with patient approval, the student can perform these skills while being directly observed by the preceptor. In some settings, getting feedback from the patient can also be helpful to the student.

Role Modeling

Preceptors serve as role models for the student. The preceptor should demonstrate respect for the student as part of the healthcare team and should expect the student to demonstrate professionalism with the clinical staff and other members of the team. The preceptor should set a positive example by demonstrating a mature approach through focused communication, sound clinical work, reliability, and high ethical standards.

STUDENT EVALUATION

The preceptor typically uses evaluation instruments provided by the academic institution. Most PA programs require a mid-term evaluation and a final evaluation. (See examples of instruments in Appendix B.) The information gathered using these evaluation instruments comes from the clinical experience and is shared with the student and with the educational program. The best evaluation methods are through direct observation, student questioning, demonstration, medical record review, student presentations, and student self-assessment.

Evaluation forms may also include sections on student's attitudes, behaviors, and interpersonal skills. The preceptor and the student should have a concluding interview to review the evaluation that will be submitted to the academic program. Discussing the clinical experience, noting the professional growth, and making suggestions for improvement are important components of this interview. It is not uncommon for the preceptor to invite the student to maintain contact and to invite future professional interactions.

CRITICAL THINKING

Teaching and learning during clinical rotations should be focused on critical thinking, sometimes called clinical reasoning. Paul and Elder, in *The Miniature Guide for Critical Thinking: Concepts and Tools,*[2] reported clinical thinking as a process of continuous improvement in a student's quality of thinking about problems. Most PA students have demonstrated critical thinking skills; they have gotten into PA school and have completed the didactic component. Therefore, they are assumed to be good "entry-level" thinkers at the start of the clinical experience. According to Weber, a preceptor cannot make a student think critically "unless the student has the desire to reach for clinical practice excellence."[3] The job of the clinical preceptor, therefore, is to encourage the student to be clear, accurate, precise, and relevant in his or her approach to clinical decision-making.

PITFALLS IN CLINICAL TEACHING

Toffler et al. discuss various pitfalls of precepting in *Family Medicine in 2001.*[4] While teaching PA students can be rewarding, there are conditions that may interfere with the process. The following list paraphrases pitfalls:

1. Over-committed and/or stressed clinicians are not good preceptor candidates. Exhaustion, irritability, and/or depression are not good traits to model to a student.
2. Over-lecturing or expecting too much in 1 day will limit the learning experience. Preceptors should not try to teach too much. One or two important concepts each day is probably plenty for the student to comprehend and retain.
3. Students do not need to observe everything the preceptor does. Passively following the preceptor will grow old for the preceptor and will be painful for the student. Other activities should be planned for the student during those times when the preceptor is occupied with other business.
4. Preceptors should not make assumptions about the PA student's knowledge. This is an important point. PA students come from varied backgrounds and experiences. Whether it is their first rotation or their last, all students present at different levels.
5. Preceptors must review the student's work. Students expect feedback, and a review is an excellent time to discuss important teaching points.
6. Preceptors should not assume that documentation by the student is adequate or appropriate. Student documentation must be reviewed for personal judgment or bias as well as for medical content and legal liability issues.
7. A preceptor should not give the student the impression that he or she would rather not have a student. If personal or professional issues interfere with precepting a student on a particular day, the preceptor should make provisions for the student to work with a colleague or a staff member for a specified period of time.

8. Steps should be taken to avoid misrepresentation. It is important both to the student and to the patient that the patient knows that the PA student is a student and not a doctor.
9. Preceptors must assess student competence. This, of course, should be discussed outside the examination room and away from the patient.
10. Preceptors should avoid subtle "put downs" of the student, particularly in front of patients or peers.
11. Preceptors should mention issues that are a source of annoyance. It is important that annoyances be discussed early and in detail.
12. Preceptors should contact the education program representatives for discussion, support, and advice.

Having PA students in the practice requires planning, orientation, effective teaching, and evaluation. It can be a rewarding, stimulating, and enjoyable experience.

REFERENCES

1. Dent JA. Teaching and learning medicine. In: Dent JA, Harden RM, eds. *A Practical Guide for Medical Teachers.* London: Churchill Livingstone; 2001: 1–10.
2. Paul R, Elder X. *The Miniature Guide for Critical Thinking: Concepts and Tools* Available at: http://www.criticalthinking.org. Accessed November 30, 2010.
3. Weber S. Promoting critical thinking in students. *J Am Acad Nurse Pract.* 2005;17(6):205–206.
4. Toffler WL, Taylor AD, Schludermann P. Pitfalls of precepting. *Fam Med.* 2001;33(10):730–731.

Chapter 11

Student Responsibilities and Guidelines

Physician assistant (PA) students look forward to the clinical phase of training, often thinking that it will be a pleasant change from the long, structured hours of classroom instruction. Instead they quickly discover that the clinical year has its own type of structure to include the daily completion of chart notes, the unpredictability of a day of patient encounters, and the stress of moving from one clinical site to another—just as they felt they were "settling in." Overall, though, students look back on their clinical year as a unique time in their life, filled with challenging and helpful patients, inspiring—though demanding—role models, and the opportunity to figure out where they best "fit" in the rapidly changing healthcare system!

The following guidelines are examples of the information provided to students regarding their role and responsibilities:[1]

STUDENT RESPONSIBILITIES TO THE PRECEPTOR, THE SITE, AND THE PATIENTS

1. The PA student should contact the preceptor 2 weeks in advance of beginning the clinical assignment to verify the arrangements.

Preceptors and their staffs want to be sure you have the information you need about clinic times, dress code, and even parking. Use this contact to ask whether there is any other information you need to know and whether they need anything from you prior to the first day, such as personal information records or results of background checks. Be certain to ask about computer access and Internet connectivity.

2. PA students are expected to maintain office hours that have been negotiated with the preceptor and communicated to office personnel. Students should realize that the scheduling of patients and the scheduling of the preceptor's time are an important consideration. PA students are expected to be sensitive to the pressure on the preceptor.

   The old adage of "go early, stay late," is apropos here. Much of the most significant communication may occur informally before or after office hours, and it is important for the PA student to be there in order not to miss it. The PA student should inform the preceptor if he or she has childcare or transportation issues; however, the program's view is that PA student should adapt her or his schedule to the clinic's schedule rather than the other way around.

3. PA students are expected to have discussions with and update the preceptor regularly on progress toward meeting the program's objectives and assignments. Scheduled meetings with the preceptor are appropriate for completion and discussion of evaluation form(s).

   The program provides information to the preceptor on required assignments and evaluation processes; however, preceptors rarely follow these guidelines closely—given their other clinical responsibilities. Preceptors may also supervise a range of students from a range of clinical programs, so they do not track the specifics of assignments or evaluation deadlines. It is the student's responsibility to keep the preceptor, and perhaps even the office staff, updated on these timelines.

4. The PA student is expected to inform the preceptor regularly of student needs. This includes identifying where the patient

"is" and "ought to be" in specific clinical requirements, patient encounters, and clinical skills.

The preceptor expects the PA student to inform her or him if the student is not able to complete required types of patient interactions. The preceptor may assign the student to work with a receptionist or scheduler, for example, to assist the student to schedule evaluation meetings.

5. The PA student is expected to show sensitivity to the wishes of patients and to be willing to share confidences or to have a student partially responsible for their care.

   Some types of patient encounters are more sensitive than others. Similarly, some patients have more experience with student involvement and may be more comfortable with it. For example, the PA student should not feel rejected if a physician or patient asks them to leave the room to discuss sensitive psychosocial issues.

6. The PA student is expected to be aware of and to apply HIPAA regulations regarding the privacy of patients' confidential information.[2]

   HIPAA rules have many implications that may not be immediately obvious to students in early phases of their clinical development. Even if a PA student received HIPAA training in the didactic phase of education, individual institutions may require the student to complete it again. Students are expected to be graciously cooperative about this.

   If a clinical rotation site uses electronic medical records, the PA student should be careful not to access the records of any patient for whom she or he is not clinically assigned.

7. PA students are expected to complete charting at the end of each day—and ideally at the completion of each patient encounter. Charts may never be removed from the clinic. Electronic medical records should be used as assigned.

   The incidence of medical errors from documentation increases with the increased time between the patient encounter and the chart note. Students should learn how to be efficient in charting and should not procrastinate. Delays also are problematic for supervising physicians, who must countersign all student records.

8. Students are expected to use technology appropriately. This includes electronic medical records, Internet access, and e-mail. Consideration of others with whom computers or computer access is shared is important.

    Some sites have designated computers for each student; others require that students share with each other or with their supervising physician. While this may create efficiency problems, it also means that each computer user becomes aware of how other users spend their time on the computer. Using breaks to access social networking sites or for online shopping is not only unacceptable but also destroys the student's credibility. Similarly, using handheld technology (e.g., PDAs such as iPhones, Blackberries) to access nonclinical information sites is not appropriate during assigned clinical hours. This includes texting and the use of Web sites such as Twitter.

9. Some preceptors assign reading lists, exams, or projects specific to their practice. These assignments should be completed along with the program's assignments.

    The best learning experiences are those related to specific encounters. Typical assignments from preceptors may include discussions about patients seen previously in the day or return patients scheduled for the following day. PA students should be prepared for in-depth discussions of these topics—even if they are not "official" assignments. Be curious!

10. PA students should be appreciative and respectful of office/clinic/hospital staff.

    While the supervising physician (and/or her/his clinical system) have agreed to volunteer as teachers, the support staff is seldom involved in this decision. The presence of a student may be viewed as a burden that creates extra work for them. Students should be aware of this possibility and should strive to allay these concerns with a helpful, cooperative attitude. Support staff hold the key to helping the student access appropriate patients and information, and staff usually introduces the student to the patients.

Students should offer to help staff when appropriate and should work at connecting with them. "Bring donuts!"

11. PA students should provide the very best care possible for the patients. Importantly, this includes saying "I don't know, I'll find out," or "I want the doctor to check this." At the same time, each student should assert his or her proven skills to the fullest.

Some medical educators have noticed that PA students are great role models for medical students in terms of saying "I don't know" or "I need someone to check on this." Supervising physicians expect to be consulted—and they also expect that the student will be prepared to engage in valuable discourse about clinical findings and problem solving.

12. If conflicts arise, students are expected to discuss the issues and to resolve them to the best of their ability. If these attempts are unsuccessful, the program's clinical coordinator or advisor expects to be notified for assistance, support, and problem solving.

Busy clinics and hospitals are full of conflict—often over scarce resources or insufficient time. Healthcare workers expect these types of conflict, and they also expect to solve them. This is particularly difficult when the issues involve strong personalities. Many students jump to the conclusion that a perceived conflict may be "about them" when actually it is a pattern of the individuals involved. If in doubt, students should check in with their clinical coordinator.

STUDENTS' RESPONSIBILITIES TO THE PROGRAM

1. Students must inform the program office of unresolved issues immediately.

Item #12 (in the previous list) discusses conflict. While conflicts are not unusual, ongoing conflicts that disrupt clinical training are of major concern. The program expects the student to initiate this contact.

2. Students must attend all orientation activities as required.

Both the program and individual clinical settings will regularly conduct orientation sessions. For the program the purpose is to provide specific information about the clinical information which may have been overstated or overwhelming in the didactic year. Examples of this include specific information about billing, coding, or a specific electronic medical record system. Institutions may conduct required sessions relating to compliance, patient safety, or new Medicare/Medicaid rules.

It is never acceptable to miss these sessions. Students with attendance issues may be placed on program probation.

3. Students must update their immunizations and background checks in compliance with institutional guidelines. Students are expected to maintain their own personal records.

Item #3 in the first section discusses the student's responsibility to become aware of and to meet professional clinical obligations. In any future medical career, PAs (and other healthcare workers) will regularly be asked to provide immunization records as part of the clinical credentialing and privileging process in institutions. Naturally, an organized and concise process for maintaining and accessing these documents is vital to both employment and safety in the healthcare field.

4. Students are expected to check e-mail every day (at least once during every 24 hours—including weekends).

Updates to clinical schedules are constant, as are returned assignments and tests. The program considers e-mail to be the "gold standard" for communication with students—students should be certain to check it regularly.

5. Students must complete electronic patient logs daily and must submit them according to the required schedule.

Just as it is important to complete charts daily, it is also important to enter and maintain patient logs in the same manner. Patient logs are certain to become a regular part of all clinician's records in the future—to be used for maintaining clinical privileges and for oversight by payers maintaining "report cards" on the providers they reimburse.

Maintaining these logs is a good habit to cultivate during clinical training.

The program uses data from patient logs to set the "required numbers" of patient encounters for each rotation. The logs are also used to guarantee that all students achieve the minimum numbers of interactions required for compliance with the program's primary care competencies.

6. Students must plan their time during each clinical rotation.

   Students should meet with their preceptors early in the rotation to verify their schedules. This is especially important if the rotation includes working away from the clinic and/or with another provider. Planning calendars should be submitted to the program regularly.

7. Students must complete assignments as required by the program and by the preceptor.

   These assignments reflect the program's expectations and quotas for competency. Specific reading, writing, and/or checklist assignments are required for each rotation. Students should make copies for their own files before submitting assignments to the program.

8. Students must complete online testing requirements as assigned. Students should ask preceptors in advance if they need consideration for dedicated time and/or space for these exams.

   Typically the program's online exams at the end of each rotation have a 24-hour window for completion. Programs do not expect students to use clinic time to log on and complete these exams. Students should contact the clinical office with any questions.

9. Students should plan for program "call-back" sessions.

   Student must complete necessary assignments (e.g., case presentations, journal club readings, reports on community education projects) ahead of time. Students should also plan to spend informal and social time with their classmates. It is important to compare notes and tell stories about clinical experiences and professional growth.

10. State and national conference attendance is a privilege, and students must be in good standing and must receive program permission in advance to attend them.

    The program encourages attendance at state, regional, and national meetings but wants to be certain that they present minimum disruption to scheduled learning experiences.

STUDENTS' RESPONSIBILITIES TO THEMSELVES

1. Students are responsible for their own clinical progress and for making their needs known to the preceptor and to the program.

    Students are expected to be assertive rather than passive in managing their clinical progress. For some students, this is a major transition from prior clinical roles where they were expected to be "followers" rather than active participants.

2. Before the clinical year begins, students should assess and develop their technological expertise to be sure it is adaptable to the clinical setting. Understanding software and computer settings (e.g., Wi-Fi and Internet access) are especially important in every clinical setting.

3. The student should schedule adequate time for readings, intensive study, written assignments/papers, and completion of electronic requirements such as patient logs.

    Some of these activities should be completed daily and others spread throughout the week. A consistent schedule is important.

4. Students should schedule weekly leisure and social time in order to maintain a healthy balance with educational responsibilities.

    Different activities work for different students. Some students need exercise; others need time for reading or time with family. Students should do what works!

5. Students should keep lines of communication open with family, support groups, their preceptors, classmates, and the program.

   Compared to the didactic year—when there is almost too much "togetherness" with classmates, the clinical year can be lonely, and students often feel isolated. Students should maintain supportive contacts and initiate conversations!

6. Students should schedule and carry out formal board preparation activities each week.

   These activities may involve the use of review books, group study sessions, or online products. Students must be certain to review the NCCPA blueprint for the PANCE exam as a study guide. The NCCPA self-assessment exam should be taken 6 to 8 weeks prior to graduation and the time remaining prior to the final exam should be used to address identified strengths and weaknesses.

REFERENCES

1. MEDEX Northwest Division of Physician Assistant Studies Physician Assistant Training Program. *Clinical Manual*, University of Washington School of Public Health and Community Medicine and the School of Medicine. Seattle, WA. 2010.
2. US Dept. of Health and Human Services. Health Information Privacy. Available at: http://www.hhs.gov/ocr/privacy/. Accessed May 21, 2010.

Chapter 12

Student Clinical Evaluations

In contrast to some other medical programs, where a culture may support "passing" a student even though they have poor performance, physician assistant (PA) programs expect preceptors to realistically evaluate students and to give them a failing grade when appropriate.

The PA clinical training culture is based on the fact that students have only 1 year of clinical training. During that year it is important to employ multiple monitoring tools (including patient logs, end of rotation exams, written assignments, and site visits). However, the evaluation of the preceptor is considered to be the most important indicator of a student's progress. For short rotations there may be only 1 evaluation; for longer rotations less complex "formative" evaluations throughout the experience may be followed by a final summative evaluation that may be used for grading a student's performance.

Some programs rely exclusively on the preceptor's assessment to determine the grade or whether a student has passed or failed. Other programs use a formula that may include all of the program components, and/or an additional assessment by the faculty advisor as well as the preceptor's evaluation. Some programs ask the preceptor to determine simply whether the student has passed or failed. Other programs use grading systems with a larger list of options including "borderline" or "exceptional performance." Evaluation forms may also provide an opportunity for the preceptor to request a verbal conference with the student's faculty advisor in order to have a more informal—but detailed—discussion.

In addition to reviewing a student's performance in a specific rotation, the cumulative student record, containing all clinical evaluations, is used by the program to evaluate a student's clinical development across the span of the clinical year.

Other evaluation tools typically used in PA programs include a pre-placement site evaluation, a site visit report, and a student evaluation of a site/preceptor (see Appendix B).

A clinical evaluation form for a PA program typically asks the preceptor to rank and/or discuss the performance or other issues in multiple areas:

1. Knowledge of Basic Medicine
   Students are expected to have a broad base of knowledge that can be recalled and related to the cases seen during the day. In addition, students should be able to readily and quickly access information as needed, using appropriate resources, publications, Web sites, and databases.

2. History-Taking Skills
   Students should be able to obtain and document a comprehensive history, to elicit important information, to follow up on specific details, and to describe findings.

3. Physical Examination Skills
   The physical exam should be thorough and logical as well as technically reliable. Technical errors are a common problem in the early phases of training and should be identified. Documentation is also a component of this skill set.

4. Knowledge/Utilization/Interpretation of Laboratory and Diagnostic Tests
   The student should demonstrate knowledge of routine and special diagnostic tests and should be able to correctly interpret the results.

5. Integrative Skills

   The ability to integrate data, identify problems and priorities, and consider additional data requirements is imperative for clinical practice.

6. Written Skills

   Write ups should be concise and orderly and should include relevant information. A key component of this skill is *prompt* completion of the medical record, allowing for a "sign-off" by the supervising physician.

7. Oral Skills

   Oral communication includes the effective, concise, organized, and complete presentation of data in the form of case summaries, hall-side consultations, and telecommunication interactions.

8. Management Skills

   Students are expected to promptly implement an agreed upon plan that has been discussed with the preceptor and to consider alternative plans and treatments, including follow-up.

9. Judgment

   Utilizing medical judgment involves timing and coordination based on data as well as the appropriate consultation with the preceptor.

10. Interaction with Patients

    Listening to patients, giving explanations, participating in discussions regarding care, and patient education are the components to be considered in evaluating patient interaction. Students should be approachable but should maintain professional boundaries.

11. Interaction with Other Health Professionals

    Cooperation and recognition of the professional roles of others are important. Knowing one's own strengths and limitations are also components of this skill.

12. Professional Behaviors

    The required behaviors for PAs include dependability, initiative, integrity, and appearance. (See Chapter 13.)

13. General Behaviors

Often the best way to address unwanted or negative behaviors is through a description of the behavior. An example of a behavioral list from a poor clinical evaluation form could include the following:

a. Incomplete work: unfinished chart work, assignments not done.

b. Absenteeism: repeated absence from activities, lateness, not available for rounds, conferences.

c. Poor attitude: negativism, chronic complaining, lack of enjoyment in work.

d. Sloppy or imprecise work: insufficient attention to quality, need to recheck database or orders.

e. Unresponsive to correction: when deficiencies are pointed out, does not correct them; makes same errors repeatedly.

f. Impracticality: impractical plans and suggestions, dangerous orders, off on tangents.

g. Inefficiency: works hard, gets nothing done.

h. Does not know what's going on: needs to be spoon fed daily orders, progress notes.

i. Timid, insecure: performance may be affected by lack of self-confidence.

j. Does not know own limitations: not cautious enough, proceeds on own without checking with appropriate person; overestimates abilities.

k. Inability to prioritize and manage multiple tasks.

l. Unable to deal with stress and complexities of the clinical situation.

m. Inappropriate use of technology: uses clinic time for personal communication/social networking/other non-clinical internet transactions.

n. Other

Programs differ in their policies about the significance of the student evaluation from the preceptor. In some programs this evaluation makes up the entire student grade.

In other programs the preceptor evaluation may be combined with other components such as an advisor's evaluation, attendance records, or grades for assignments—including electronic patient logs and written papers, and grades for end-of-rotation exams. Students are generally required to repeat rotations for which they do not receive a passing grade.

The preceptor is generally expected to discuss the evaluation with the student. In the final/summative evaluation for a clinical experience, the preceptor can provide additional feedback to the student and may also wish to receive feedback for her/himself about the student's experience. Most preceptors are familiar with this process from multiple similar experiences with medical students and residents. The summative evaluation form may include a place for both the preceptor's and the student's signatures.

REFERENCE

Materials in this chapter are derived from conversations with Ruth Ballweg (University of Washington) and Michael Goodwin (A.T. Still University), March 2010.

Chapter 13

Professional Behavior

Professionalism is hard to define specifically; we usually know when we see it yet recognize when it is not present. This broad concept, for some, is synonymous with ethical behavior. Many of us think of professionalism in terms of specifics such as a clinician's appearance, of communication skills, of being culturally competent, of general civility, or even of simply being on time. Of course, it is all of those things and more. As an introduction, some obvious examples of non-professional behavior are listed here:

1. A male PA abruptly enters into an examination room where a female patient is waiting. The PA says, "Hi Darlin', I'm Dr. X. Don't mind the little bit of blood on my lab coat, I promise not to lose my next patient. So, what are you here for?"
2. An attending physician in a clinic says to a new PA student: "You're here officially under my supervision, but I trust you've learned much of what you need to know before you got here, so I'll trust you to be on your own. You don't need to bother me. Just make sure that you always code on the chart for the maximum service for the diagnosis. You don't need to actually do all those things, but for us it's better accounting."

Looking at these extreme examples, how many unprofessional behaviors can you spot? In the first situation, it was not mentioned that the

PA knocked before entering. He has inappropriately identified himself as a doctor. He greets the patient in an inappropriate way. He makes what, to many patients, would be an upsetting attempt at humor. He has not changed out of a soiled lab coat. He has not read the chart that contains the chief complaint of the patient. In the second situation, the PA student is there to learn and to be supervised. It is inappropriate for her/him to be left on their own without consultation, ideally directly, with the person charged with their supervision. The PA student is, therefore, doing work that will be billed by the attending physician. Billing should always directly reflect what is done; to do otherwise is not only unprofessional but also fraudulent.

In this chapter we examine the specific components of professional behavior of both the student (and future) PA and of the supervising physician in relation to the PA student.

Also, by way of introduction, we should mention that the concept of professionalism is relatively new. At one time, anyone with knowledge and skills put into the service of others was considered a professional.[1] In health care, that idea became far more 3-dimensional when a humanism project was begun by The American Board of Internal Medicine. That project, in turn, led to Project Professionalism in the mid-1980s.[2] In this work, the importance of ethical behavior came to the fore. Over the years, professionalism has become a constant, albeit complex, part of PA training and standards. While for the physician the focus has been on relations primarily with the patient, for the PA the focus is also on relationships with other professionals, particularly physicians, as well as to the whole healthcare system and society at large.

The National Commission on Certification of Physician Assistants, NCCPA, through the NCCPA Foundation, put out a guide, *Concepts in PA Excellence: Exploring Ethics, a Guide for Facilitators* in 2006.[3] It contains guidelines for "Ethical Conduct for the Physician Assistant Profession." These are excellent guideposts, and video case studies for discussion are included. Similarly, the book *Ethics and Professionalism: A Guide for the Physician Assistant*[4] provides a comprehensive view that includes many excellent case studies exploring ethical issues, the proper handling of which leads to true professionalism.

The tenets of professionalism are also tightly defined by state licensing bodies in the area of supervision. While the concept of supervision does not mean that the supervising physician must always be present with the PA or direct every aspect of PA-provided care, the requirements of supervision may vary by state. The physician–PA interactions should be considered professional, no matter how the physician is supervising the PA.[5]

Often absent from discussions about professionalism are the issues that may arise out of the "business of medicine."[6] As a professional, the PA may think that referral to a specialist is important, yet a managed-care contract may restrict this. A physician's practice might own various ancillary services or equipment, such as diagnostic imaging equipment, and physicians may encourage their PAs to always refer these particular services. A PA might see "defensive medicine" practiced where a plethora of tests that he or she does not believe are needed are ordered to protect the business. In these types of dilemmas, black or white answers to what the professional PA needs to do may not be clear, but recognizing them and drawing on a collective set of professional guideposts is vital for the physician or PA supervising the PA student.

For our purposes we assume that core clinical knowledge and an ability to discern new developments in clinical knowledge through the application of evidence-based practice are the starting points upon which all parts of professionalism and effective health care are based.

COMPONENT PARTS OF PROFESSIONALISM

Professionalism is complex and has many components. In this section some of the key elements and related skills are examined in more detail.

Self-Knowledge

An often overlooked foundation of true professionalism is knowing and understanding one's preferred way of being in the world.

The nature/nurture controversy (i.e., which characteristics are inborn and genetically and physiologically linked and which result from our experience in the world) has abated. Most research shows that we are a fairly even combination of both. Regardless, if we don't know ourselves, how can we best know, understand, and interact with others?

Why is this important? First, if a person is very organized and always on time, it may be a challenge to professionally deal with a patient or a PA student being supervised who is disorganized or who comes in late. Similarly, if a person is naturally uncomfortable with conflict and must interact with combative patients or people in the office who are overly aggressive, understanding this tendency may be the key for successful professional interaction. Many instruments have been developed to help with this self-analysis; the Myers-Briggs Type Indicator and the DISC instruments are among the most commonly used. These assessments can be taken online and can be trusted to provide thoroughly researched, valid, and reliable profiles. The results can help identify areas for awareness and focus (not necessarily change), to better assess the different styles of those being mentored and/or treated as well.

Positive Interpersonal Communication

It seems self-evident that a successful healthcare practitioner needs to be able to display positive interpersonal communication skills. We know from the literature, for example, that malpractice suits are often correlated inversely with the communication skills of the practitioner rather than the commission of actual medical errors.[7] In other words, the physician who genuinely listens, understands, supports, and truly cares about the patient is far less likely to face malpractice litigation.

Positive communication integrates many skills like demonstrating attending behaviors, using questions and paraphrasing, and sharing decision-making, and it may include conflict resolution. Positive communication is timely and needs to occur within a culturally aware and appropriate context. Each of these elements is integral to the development and ultimate success of the developing PA, and the supervising physician needs to observe them, break them down individually, and give the person or people being mentored specific feedback.

Good interpersonal behavior begins with focused listening. Often referred to as *active listening*, this ability focuses on listening for meaning both verbally and nonverbally. The nonverbal element relates to picking up gestures, sounds, and interjections that extend beyond the words expressed. It also includes acknowledging what the patient is saying by paraphrasing it back in terms of facts and feelings. For the PA, good interpersonal behavior begins with a positive introduction when first meeting the patient. This meeting cannot be contrived; it implies feeling comfortable and putting the patient or client at ease with body language that expresses real interest. This initial communication continues with appropriate open and closed questions. Closed questions, such as "Where does it hurt?" have specific answers that the clinician needs to help diagnose and treat the patient. Open questions, like "How has this affected your life?" call for a broader response and often reveal both expanded facts and feelings. Paraphrasing without parroting responses from a patient shows that the PA has listened and understands; it also provides a forum in which the patient can expand and clarify answers.

Integrity/Dependability

Integrity implies dependability in professional behavior. It refers to organizational skills, proper preparation, punctuality, and appearance. Integrity also melds with positive communication in the softer, but equally important, actions of showing respect and compassion for others, as well as tolerance for the behaviors of others. Although these may be the most obvious of skills beyond positive communication, it becomes clear when they are not present. Many of us have waited inordinate amounts of time in a doctor's office or for other appointments with professionals. Physicians and PAs alike can get backed up, can have emergencies arise, or can have other events that put them behind in their appointment schedule. However, making sure that patients are aware of the issues and perhaps offering to reschedule shows respect for and understanding of the needs of a patient.

Similarly, taking the time to appear neat, clean, and professional is vital. Feedback for the supervised PA in these areas is important.

As a professional displaying integrity, the PA is expected to be a lifelong learner. Much of the information taught in school will be replaced by newer knowledge, tests, and techniques, often within a very short period of time. Patients or clients are often very educated, and they have often been exposed to advertising with which they may assume the practitioner is familiar. Reading peer-reviewed journals and keeping up with the changes in practice is also a mark of integrity. Reading, understanding, and synthesizing evidence-based knowledge relies on the peer-review process plus the use of analytical skills. In a previous chapter we discussed the importance of testing the PA student by asking the student to present or otherwise display this professional skill of literature review.

Yet another element of professional integrity is related to giving back or providing service to the community. With a busy practice this is often difficult, but some volunteering, whether using medical skills or in other arenas, is something one typically observes in highly professional and successful individuals. With the discipline necessary to become a PA, the potential for leadership is large. Participating in projects where the PA can make use of this characteristic adds both to the community and to personal quality of life and should be encouraged by the physician or PA supervisor.

Cultural Competence

Understanding the local culture of typical patients may be the key to effectively providing treatment in a professional manner. This awareness of thoughts, communications, actions, beliefs, and customs is derived from one or more factors, including race, ethnicity, gender, marital status, age, sexual orientation, veteran status, national origin, disability, religious affiliation, and socio-economic status. Cultural competence is "a set of congruent behaviors, attitudes and policies that come together in a system, agency, or among professionals that enables effective work in cross-cultural situations."[8]

Without a good understanding of a patient's culture, the potential for behavioral misinterpretations arises. For example, in many western cultures, good eye contact is considered important. As a result, a PA with eyes downcast, who never establishes eye contact, may convey a depressed or disinterested affect. However, in some cultures, averting the eyes may simply be a way of showing respect. In other words, gestures in one culture may have very different meanings in another. In some cultures a female would never be comfortable being seen by a male practitioner.

The goals of cultural competence include both knowledge and attitudes. They begin with appreciating the differences that exist within and across cultural groups and the need to avoid negative stereotyping. Like other areas of professionalism, a great deal has been written about cultural competence. One of the most common models used in health care is the Kleinman explanatory model.[9] Kleinman et al. discuss the differences between disease and illness. For example, a patient complains of pain, which is later diagnosed as chronic cholecystitis, and his gall bladder is subsequently surgically removed. The patient's condition fails to improve significantly. Ultimately, the patient comes from a culture that believes in being "hexed" or "bewitched." He believes that this is the cause of his "illness" and that this "sickness" can only be removed by removing the curse. The physician calls in an indigenous healer from the patient's culture, a ceremony is performed, and the patient fully recovers. We can often cure the illness but the culturally competent PA also needs to acknowledge the sickness.

A model to practice cultural competence used in health care called LEARN has been created by Berlin and Fowkes.[10] It focuses on the need for culturally appropriate communication. The acronym LEARN stands for Listening, Eliciting responses, Assessing, Recommending, and Negotiating. *Listening and eliciting responses* corresponds to "active listening" described above. It requires the practitioner to make sure that an interpreter is available as needed, that open questions are asked, and that answers are heard without interruption. This model emphasizes the importance of having the patient talk about the expected results of the visit. *Assessing* goes beyond medical testing and includes consideration of problems in the patient's life that may impact health and health behaviors. *Recommendations* include the diagnosis and the treatment plan. Finally, *negotiations* create agreement between the practitioner and patient so that both are invested in the options agreed upon.

Functioning Under Stress

Virtually everyone who works in health care operates under stress. From the pioneering work of Hans Selye[11] and later researchers, we understand that, while stress is normal (and can be beneficial), stress can become "*dis*tress." Physiologically, humans deal with stress through a "fight or flight" or "general adaptation" mechanism, followed by rest and recalibration to a lower level of stress. However, often there is no time for rest or recovery as we move from one crisis to another. The stress then accumulates and can impact everything from sleep patterns to digestion to immune responses to blood pressure. What does this have to do with professionalism?

The PA who does not recognize stress or does nothing to deal with it, risks becoming physically ill or emotionally drained, both of which impact professional patient care. Formerly, "baptism by fire" was an acceptable practice imposed on physician interns, often including 24- or 36-hour shifts. Studies have demonstrated that this significantly damaged the quality of patient care and could lead to serious medical errors.[12,13] Getting enough sleep is an important first step in remaining "professionally fit."

Dealing with stress includes keeping healthy in a variety of ways. Self-knowledge, positive interpersonal communication, and integrity, by themselves, can lower stress levels. Regular exercise and community involvement can also help. Self-care may include spending short periods per day doing slow deep breathing, positive visualizations, yoga, and meditation. Becoming aware of personal stressors and learning the many ways to cope with them, should be actively pursued by every PA.[14]

CONCLUSION

The truly professional PA is an individual who actively seeks self-knowledge and who learns and practices positive communication, who understands patient concerns, and who becomes culturally competent. Professional PAs display integrity and are dependable; they have a positive attitude toward patients and colleagues. With the patient, they honor the individuality of each person seen. With colleagues, they learn that they are a part of a complex team of healthcare workers. The ultimate professional is what Greenleaf called a "servant leader"[15]: a role model with caring and ethical behavior that uses a holistic approach to individual needs. Pursuit and practice of such characteristics will lead the future PA to become a consummate professional.

REFERENCES

1. Parsons T. *The Social System.* Glencoe, IL: The Free Press; 1951.
2. American Board of Internal Medicine (ABIM). *Project Professionalism.* Philadelphia, PA: American Board of Internal Medicine; 1994.
3. Lombardo P, Cohn R, Goldgar C, eds. *Concepts in PA Excellence: Exploring Ethics– A Guide to Facilitators.* Atlanta, GA: NCCPA Foundation; 2006.
4. Cassidy BA, Blessing JD. *Ethics and Professionalism: A Guide for the Physician Assistant.* Philadelphia, PA: E.A. David Co.; 2008.
5. American Academy of Physician Assistants. *State Law Issues: Supervision of PAs: Access and Excellence in Patient Care.* 2010. Available at : http://www.aapa.org/images/stories/IssueBriefs/State%20Law%20Issues/PA%20Supervision%20-%202010.pdf. Accessed February 15, 2011.
6. Ballweg R, Stolberg S, Sullivan EM. *Physician Assistant: A Guide to Clinical Practice,* 3rd ed. Philadelphia, PA: Saunders; 2003, p. 121.
7. Hickson GB, Jenkins DA. Identifying and addressing communication failures as a means of reducing unnecessary malpractice claims. *NC Med J.* 2007;68(5):362–364.
8. Cross T, Barzon B, Dennis K, Isaacs M. *Towards a Culturally Competent System of Care: A Monograph on Effective Services for Minority Children Who Are Severely Emotionally Disturbed.* Vol. 1. Washington, DC: Georgetown University Child Development Center; 1989.
9. Kleinman A, Eisenberg L, Good B. Culture, illness and care: Clinical lessons from anthropologic and cross-cultural research. *Ann Internal*

Med. 88(1978): 251–258. (Reprinted in *Focus* 2006;4 [Winter]:140–149, American Psychiatric Association.)

10. Berlin EA, Fowkes WC. Teaching framework for cross-cultural care: Application in family practice. *West J Med.* 1983;139(6):934–938.

11. Selye H. *Stress Without Distress.* Philadelphia, PA: Lippincott, Wilkins & Williams; 1973.

12. Drazen JM. Awake and informed. *N Eng JMed.* 2004;351(18):1884.

13. Landrigan CP, Rothschild JM, Cronin JW, Kaushal R, Burdick E, Katz JT, et al. Effect of reducing interns' work hours on serious medical errors in intensive care units. *N Eng J Med.* 2004;351(18):1838–1848.

14. Sapolsky RM. *Why Zebras Don't Get Ulcers: An Updated Guide to Stress, Stress Related Diseases, and Coping.* 2nd ed. New York, NY: WH Freeman; 1998.

15. Sipe S L, Frick D M. *The Seven Pillars of Servant Leadership*, Mahwah, NJ: Paulist Press; 2009.

Supervising Physician Assistants

Chapter 14

Hiring a Physician Assistant

There are nearly 80,000 trained physician assistants (PAs), with more than 5000 new graduates entering the job market each year.[1] Physician assistants practice in nearly every clinical setting in the American medical system. Accordingly, PAs work in environments that include a solo-physician practice, multi-physician practice, or institutions/corporations. The employment status of the PA is most often as an employee, while some work as a self-employed contractor. This chapter will outline a common-sense process related to the hiring of a PA.

The suggested steps for hiring a PA include the following:

1. Assessment of the organization/practice culture
2. Evaluation of billing/productivity systems
3. Development of a job description
4. Consideration of a supervision/quality assurance model
5. Determination of employment status
6. Development of a compensation plan
7. Consideration of the applicable state PA practice act
8. Developing an employment contract
9. Finding a PA
10. Making an offer

ASSESSMENT OF THE ORGANIZATION/ PRACTICE CULTURE

Whether the medical practice is ready for a PA must be determined at the outset. Are the supervising physicians favorable to supervising a PA? Is the support staff familiar with the role and scope of a PA? Has the organization/practice had experience with a PA? All of these factors affect the success or failure of a PA working on the supervising physician–PA team. The supervising physician(s) should be willing to be supportive of a PA. Difficulties arise when an employee physician is forced to supervise a PA. The job description of the employed or contracted physician should include PA supervision. The physician owner or principal owner is commonly in favor of hiring a PA because of the direct financial advantages and quality-of-life benefits. The support staff is also important to the PA's success. Administrative personnel, nursing staff, and medical technicians often benefit from an orientation or in-service presentation that educates them on the role, scope, and elements of general supervision and clinical involvement of the PA. The concept of physician services delivered by a nonphysician can be confusing to the staff and patients. Openly reviewing the concept of the physician–PA team facilitates the integration of the PA as a medical partner.[2] The first PA in a practice may experience an occasional obstacle or barrier. Some of these issues can be anticipated by predetermining ways in which the physician and the PA can resolve identified obstacles and barriers. Communication with and consistency in message to staff, vendors, and patients as it relates to the physician–PA team is paramount.

EVALUATION OF BILLING/PRODUCTIVITY SYSTEMS

Measuring the efficacy of any medical treatment or intervention is key to the financial success of any practice. It is equally important to measure the financial productivity and/or impact of the PA. The PA delivers physician services with general physician supervision.[3] As described in Chapter 5, the revenue generated by the PA can approach that of a physician in many settings. Considering the ways in which the revenue and expenses might be tracked will foster evidenced-based decision making as it relates to PA utilization and compensation on an ongoing basis. Chapter 5 provided examples of profit and loss statements that require specific information from various sources.

Revenue can be viewed from the perspective of both gross revenue and billable accounts receivable. Gross revenue is simply what is billed by the PA (i.e., prevailing charges). This number, however, may not equal the accounts receivable. It could be more useful to track the actual revenue collected compared to actual charges. Ambiguity can arise between the economic value of the PA to the practice when charges do not correlate to actual collections. Clearly, if the generated charges do not result in actual collected revenue, the long-term economic contribution of the PA is significantly diminished. Communication and transparency with regard to the economic value of the PA to the practice can drive a number of favorable behaviors. Sharing a financial statement with the PA can be enlightening and empowering. The PA is often not aware of the actual revenue, expenses, and contribution their clinical practice generates. Including the PA as a professional and partner, to an appropriate degree, in the financial goals of the organization can result in improved revenue generation, coding quality, and the reduction of overhead expenses.

JOB DESCRIPTION

Defining "who, what, when, where, and why" as it relates to the PA's clinical practice, is an essential part of a well-written PA job description. The job description should outline the general position requirements, special skills, and other essential attributes regarding the PA's performance of clinical duties. The American Academy of Physician Assistants (AAPA) suggests that the job description reflect the style of the practice and the supervising physician while detailing which patients should be treated, where the PA will work, and whether call duty is required.[2] Clear descriptions also set clear expectations that avoid future problems.

The PA's job description is a living document that should be periodically reviewed and updated. In many states, the job description is used or required as a supporting document for the practice plan or delegation agreement with the PA regulatory board. The job description should not include the details of compensation, quality assurance, or specific details of clinical duties. These specifics should be detailed in a delegation agreement or practice plan.

A publication by the AAPA entitled *Program to Practice: A Guide to the Physician Assistant Profession,* is extremely valuable and widely available.

SUPERVISION AND QUALITY ASSURANCE

Physician supervision is a dynamic relationship that thrives in an environment of a high level of trust, open communication, and empowered delegation.[4] Adverse outcomes may often be avoided when the aforementioned characteristics are practiced by the supervising physician–PA team (see Chapter 15). All state laws and practice acts require the supervising physician to be available to the PA by some communication means that can include telephone, radio, or other electronic methods.[5,6] Only a handful of states do not allow for remote supervision.[5,6]

Because the PA practices within the scope of the supervising physician, it is important to thoughtfully determine the skill level of the PA. A new graduate or a PA new to the practice setting will probably require more oversight and mentoring initially. Creating even the most basic professional development plan that outlines the clinical education, experience, skills, and knowledge along with a plan to address any shortfall or gaps is a sound practice. A professional development plan could also be used as a basis for compensation or for future performance appraisals.

The seminal work of the Institute of Medicine, *Crossing the Quality Chasm,* has stimulated quality assurance and performance improvement initiatives that have pervaded health care and medicine. Considering how the PA will be supervised is a requirement for all delegation agreements and practice plans. This requirement clearly aligns well with the concepts of quality assurance. The supervising physician should follow the requirements of the applicable PA practice act; however, the concept of randomly reviewing or cosigning encounters after the fact may not achieve the desired end state of ensuring or creating the highest quality outcome. One option is to adopt a conditional measure or evidenced-based outcome quality assurance program that generates greater actionable changes in how health care is delivered by the physician–PA team.

EMPLOYMENT STATUS

A PA can be hired as an employee or retained as a subcontractor. Generally, however, the PA is hired as an employee. The employer can be the supervising physician, a multi-physician specialty corporation/entity, or a general healthcare corporation. The supervising solo-physician model is often the most informal but is becoming less common in the marketplace. Multi-specialty physician groups and healthcare corporations appear to have the greatest economies of scale and seem to benefit most from the contribution of PAs.[7,8] In certain specialties, the PA is best utilized as a non-employee or "1099" contractor. A PA in this capacity must meet the requirements published by the Internal Revenue Service. This status is seen more commonly in surgical specialties where the PA bills through a corporation as a surgical first assistant. A key in either setting is to make sure the billing requirements are well understood in order to maximize the actual collected revenue.[9]

COMPENSATION PLAN

The standard elements of PA compensation include salary, medical insurance, dental insurance, disability insurance, and retirement/401K. Additionally, common benefits may include a performance bonus, reimbursement for licenses, registrations, continuing medical education, paid time off for medical education, and professional memberships and/or dues. The largest part of the cost of hiring a PA is the salary. This aspect of compensation is usually the greatest point of negotiation before, during, and after the offer to hire has been extended. A key concept, as it relates to cash compensation, is the degree to which the salary is tied to profitability, production, or performance. A plan should be outlined with regard to how a PA will grow into her or his role in the practice. If the goal is to develop a partnership with the PA, creating a compensation plan that recognizes experience, performance, and tenure can create a team that delivers high-quality health care. One method for achieving this goal is to develop a plan or program that includes "at risk" compensation. This "at risk" compensation is not guaranteed but is based on measurable objectives that are reliably produced and contributes favorably to the practice or patient care. Adding an "at risk" component to a compensation plan can be useful for the new graduate who is developing into a more experienced clinician. This can be a win–win approach in that the practice or entity is able to hire a new graduate at a lower salary in consideration of their experience while later adding "at risk" compensation as value is added through demonstrated measurable impact.

The AAPA is an outstanding source for identifying the salary ranges and compensation of PAs, whether experienced or newly graduated. This information can be found at www.aapa.org. There is fee-based service or general salary information available under the "Data and Statistics" tab.

PHYSICIAN ASSISTANT PRACTICE ACT AND LAW

Understanding the PA practice act is essential to avoiding unfavorable interactions with the state regulatory board. Special attention should be paid to the requirements of supervision, the scope of practice, and the requirements for prescribing or dispensing medications. Both the PA and the supervising physician should read and familiarize themselves with all the aspects related to supervision and practice. Follow-up review of the practice act and related regulations as they change is strongly suggested.

EMPLOYMENT CONTRACT

The employment contract can be useful for both the hiring entity and the PA. A contract should be reviewed by legal counsel to make sure it follows the employment laws of the state. A compensation package and job description can be referenced as part of this document. In most cases, the employment contract outlines the terms and conditions of employment, terms and condition of termination, noncompete clauses, and malpractice coverage. Because of the importance of this employment contract, it would be advisable to employ an attorney to assist in its creation.

FINDING A PHYSICIAN ASSISTANT AND MAKING THE OFFER

A PA can be recruited from a number of sources. The standard approaches include running an advertisement (e.g., in a newspaper or professional journal or on a Web site), contracting with an agency, working with a PA program in the area, or recruiting from another practice. Any of these approaches can be effective. Key aspects include doing the prehiring work as it relates to practice or company preparations for the inclusion of a PA on the team. Secondly, personnel or administrative issues should be addressed. These include policies, job descriptions, and/or compensation plans. Lastly, once PA applicants are identified, they should be interviewed. If at all possible, the inclusion of a PA in the hiring process proves useful in that it adds credibility and perspective to the recruitment initiative.

REFERENCES

1. American Academy of Physician Assistants (AAPA). *2009 AAPA Physician Assistant Census Report: List of Tables and Subject Index.* Alexandria, VA: American Academy of Physician Assistants; 2009.
2. AAPA Web site. Hiring a PA. Available at: http://www.aapa.org/images/stories/Advocacy-issue-briefs/hiring_transitional_6-09.pdf. Accessed December 31, 2009.
3. AAPA Web site. Compendium of physician assistants: Introduction. Available at: http://www.aapa.org/gandp/state-law-intro.html. Accessed May 10, 2007.
4. NCCPA. Key success factors for PA–physician teams. *NCCPA Best Practices.* Duluth, GA: National Commission on the Certification of Physician Assistants Foundation; 2007:1–3.

5. AAPA Web site. Guidelines for state regulation of physician assistants. Available at: http://www.aapa.org/gandp/statoregguidelines.html. Accessed May 10, 2007.

6. AAPA Web site. Summary of state laws for physician assistants. Available at: http://www.aapa.org/gandp/statelaw.html. Accessed May 10, 2007.

7. Gans DN. Why nonphysician providers? *MGMA e-connexion.* 2005;5(10):25–27. Available at: http://www3.mgma.com/articles/index.cfm?fuseaction=detail.main&articleID=13613. Accessed May 10, 2007.

8. Vuletich M. Crunching numbers: Medium, large practices might make better use of NPPs than small practices. *MGMA e-connexion.* 2006(97). Available at: http://www.mgma.com/pm/article.aspx?id=450. Accessed May 10, 2007.

9. Nicoletti B. How to bill for services performed by nonphysician practitioners. *Fam Practice Manage.* 2006;13(5):45.

Chapter 15

Legal Aspects of Clinical Supervision

Legally, physician assistant (PA) practice is governed by a broad range of institutional, state and federal policies, rules, regulations, laws, and court decisions. At the institutional level, for example, hospital by-laws may specify PA activities and required levels of supervision. State practice acts regulate PA practice through laws and regulations. More liberal states may provide broad supervisory powers to the physician. More conservative states may be more specific in their language regarding supervision and may include details of chart review, "on-site" supervision, and remote-site practice. Federal rules and regulations are typically about reimbursement—including authorization of care—or access to specific pharmaceuticals such as narcotics.

BACKGROUND AND BASIC PRINCIPLES

Describing the historical context for PA practice, Younger et al. say that PAs:

> arrived on the health care scene during the late 1960's, a time when the American Medical Association (AMA) and the American Hospital Association (AHA) were questioning the licensure practices for all health

professionals. Within these organizations, physician-members, hospitals, and other health care professionals increasingly expressed concern that existing licensure laws posed significant barriers to educational advancement, effective delegation of tasks and innovative use of health care personnel particularly non-physician providers.[1]

A series of conferences at Duke University were held to discuss the regulation of PAs. Dr. E. Harvey Estes—one of the founders of the Duke PA Program—advocated for the "legal recognition of PAs under the license of their employing physician" to assure a "dynamic balance between a doctor and an employed PA."[2] Legal recognition of PAs under the licensure of their employing physician was envisioned as allowing more freedom and flexibility than an independent licensure law. This view of the legal Physician–PA relationship served—and continues to serve—as the basis for PA practice today.

While some physicians may feel that this relationship and PA supervision requirements are onerous, most physicians value this feature of PA practice and view it as an issue of quality and physician leadership. This arrangement is also similar to the types of supervision experienced by all physicians at the various levels of their training as medical students, residents, and fellows.

At the Duke Conferences, model legislation was drafted which described a system of state regulation combined with a delegatory process at the individual physician–PA level. The conferences recommended a 2-stage process:

1. State recognition of PAs through the state medical regulatory body, which would regulate broad aspects of the PA profession such as qualification and examination requirements for certification, applications by supervising physicians to utilize PAs and disciplinary actions against PAs.
2. Continued delineation of the individual PA's scope of practice in accordance with the medical tasks delegated by the supervising physician, who would remain liable for PA-provided patient care.[3]

SCOPE OF PRACTICE

The concept of "scope of practice" refers both to a definition of the range of tasks that a PA may legally perform and also to the extent and nature of physician supervision required for the performance of these tasks. While a wide range of regulations of supervision exists across states, the current Model Practice Act of the American Academy of Physician Assistants (AAPA) describes supervision in the following way:

> Supervision shall be continuous but shall not be construed as necessarily requiring the physical presence of the supervising physician at the time and place that the services are rendered.
>
> It is the obligation of each team of physician(s) and physician assistant(s) to ensure that the physician assistant's scope of practice is identified; that delegation of medical tasks is appropriate to the physician assistant's level of competence; that the relationship of, and access to, the supervising physician is defined; and that a process for evaluation of the physician assistant's performance is established.[4]

Language regarding the scope of practice states practice acts rarely spell out specific requirements for day-to-day activities such as chart review; however, a requirement that a written plan be developed and remain on file in the clinic may be in place. Such plans might include a specified number of charts that must be reviewed each week or month, or a plan might specify that patients in certain categories with specific conditions (e.g., infants or patients with sudden onset of chest pain) be reviewed by the physician. Typically, chart review is more frequent for new graduates and/or new employees than for more experienced or more senior PAs. More specific chart review and/or cosignature requirements in inpatient settings are typically spelled out in hospital by-laws or other policies.

"Availability" and "responsibility" are key features of the supervision of PAs, although they are rarely spelled out in detail. A provision for the designation of an alternate supervising physician is usually clear, and in some states all members of a legally constituted group practice may serve as alternate supervisors for the PAs in their group. Essentially the requirement is that the physician (or alternate) be readily available and easy to contact on a 24/7 basis. Telecommunication is commonly accepted as a mechanism for supervision.

PHYSICIAN ASSISTANTS AS AGENTS OF THE PHYSICIAN

Physician assistants are seen as agents of the supervising physician.

> With slight variations in language, the provisions in state PA practice laws regarding physician supervision generally provide that the supervising physician ultimately retains full professional and legal responsibility for the performance of the PA and the care and treatment of patients.[5]

The AAPA's Model Practice Act describes this role of "agent." Physician assistants practice medicine with physician supervision. Physician assistants may perform those duties and responsibilities, including the ordering, prescribing and dispensing, and administration of drugs and medical devices that are delegated by their supervising physician(s).

Physician assistants may provide any medical service that is delegated by the supervising physician when the service is within the PA's skills, forms a component of the physician's scope of practice, and is provided with supervision. A PA may perform a task outside the scope of practice of the supervising physician as long as the supervising physician has adequate training, oversight skills, and supervisory and referral arrangements to ensure competent provision of the service by the PA.

Physician assistants may pronounce death and may authenticate with their signature any form that may be authenticated by a physician's signature.

Physician assistants shall be considered the agents of their supervising physicians in the performance of all practice-related activities including, but not limited to, the ordering of diagnostic, therapeutic, and other medical services.[6]

In inpatient settings PAs regularly write orders for medical procedures and medications. This process was tested in the late 1970s when members of the Washington State Nurses Association challenged the authority of PAs to write medical orders. In a defining case for PA practice, the Washington Supreme Court upheld the regulations allowing this practice saying that it was "in accordance with the legislative intent of the PA practice statute," that is, that PAs are agents of their supervising physicians and therefore PA orders effectively emanate from the physician.[7,8]

LIMITS ON NUMBERS OF PHYSICIAN ASSISTANTS SUPERVISED

State PA practice acts place limits on the numbers of PAs that can be supervised by a single physician; however, there are seldom limitations on the *total* numbers of mid-level practitioners (e.g., PAs and nurse practitioners). The numbers may vary from state to state, and sometimes different limitations are specified for certain practice settings.

Ideally the practice act allows exceptions based on special requests and appeals. A major consideration is often whether or not the patients are institutionalized (e.g., correctional or long-term care facilities), where it is easier to monitor patient outcomes. In these cases, larger numbers of PAs per supervising physician may be approved.

THE SUPERVISING PHYSICIAN

Physician assistants can only be supervised by physicians who are licensed in the state where the PA is practicing. The physician must not have a restricted license—although in the event of an exception to this, the PA has the same practice restrictions as the supervising physician. For example, a physician receiving treatment in a monitored treatment program that is still allowed to remain in his/her community for practice, would not be able to utilize his/her PA to prescribe medications that are forbidden to him/her.

The supervising physician must maintain a written agreement with the PA—termed either a "practice plan" or a "job description" by most licensing boards. According to the AAPA Model Practice Act,

> The agreement must state that the physician will exercise supervision over the physician assistant in accordance with this act and any rules adopted by the board and will retain professional and legal responsibility

for the care rendered by the physician assistant. The agreement must be signed by the physician and the physician assistant and updated annually. The agreement must be kept on file at the practice site and made available to the board upon request.[9]

Table 15-1 is a "Best Practices" checklist for the administrative supervision of PAs. Physicians should be well informed about the state's PA practice act, should annually update the practice plan or job description,

Table 15–1 Physician Supervision of Physician Assistants Best Administrative Practices

1. State PA Practice
   a. Have on file.
   b. Review with each PA at employment.
   c. Receive updates from PA as they are approved.

2. PA Job Description/Practice Plan
   a. Review and sign with each PA at employment.
   b. Review and update annually at each performance review.
   c. Forward to appropriate HR/Medical Staff Offices.

3. Hospital By-Laws/Privileges
   a. Maintain an up-to-date copy of hospital by-laws including sections covering the delegation to PAs.
   b. Monitor updates as they occur.

4. Encourage PA membership/involvement in PA organizations.
   a. Charge PA with updating physician(s) on changes in regulations or policies (e.g., reimbursement).
   b. Charge PA with updating administrative staff on relevant changes in policies (e.g., reimbursement, approved authorizations, etc.).

5. Develop an internal chart review plan depending on the experience and learning goals of the PA and of the practice team.

6. Regularly assign reading/research/professional development activities.

and should rely on the PA to update the physician and the clinic's or institution's administration on regulatory changes in PA practice.

PHYSICIAN LIABILITY

With slight variations in language, the provisions in state PA practice laws regarding physician supervision generally provide that "the supervising physician ultimately retains full professional and legal responsibility for the performance of the PA and the care and treatment of patients."[10]

Because the supervising physician is always legally responsible for the PA's patient care, the physician is also liable for the PA's actions. According to the *PA Legal Handbook:*

> While the most important statutory and/or regulatory provisions pertaining to physician supervision outline specific supervisory requirements and responsibilities, another significant provision in this area addresses physician liability. Because of the dependent nature of the PA profession, all state PA statutes place liability for PA negligence in providing medical services on the supervising physician; such liability however, is shared by the PA.[11]

For this reason, malpractice coverage for PAs—although available separately—is most often carried as a "rider" on the physician's malpractice insurance or as a part of an institutional policy.

CONCLUSION

While PA supervision may seem daunting when described on paper, physicians—and physician organizations—see these supervisory practices and requirements as a major strength of the profession. As Dr. Estes said, it represents the "dynamic balance between a doctor and an employed PA."[2]

REFERENCES

1. Younger P, Conner C, Cartwright K, Kole S, Forsyth J. *Physician Assistant Legal Handbook: Aspen Law Center.* Gaithersburg, MD: Aspen Publishers; 1997, p. 63.

2. Estes EH. The PA experiment after 25 years: What we have learned. *J Am Acad Physician Assist.* 1992;716.

3. Younger P, Conner C, Cartwright K, Kole S, Forsyth J. *Physician Assistant Legal Handbook: Aspen Law Center.* Gaithersburg, MD: Aspen Publishers; 1997, p. 65.

4. American Academy of Physician Assistants (AAPA). Model Practice Act. Available at: http://www.aapa.org/advocacy-and-practice-resources/state-advocacy/490-model-state-legislation. Accessed June 30, 2010.

5. Younger P, Conner C, Cartwright K, Kole S, Forsyth J. *Physician Assistant Legal Handbook: Aspen Law Center.* Gaithersburg, MD: Aspen Publishers; 1997, p. 76.

6. AAPA Model Practice Act. 2009. Available at: http://www.aapa.org/advocacy-and-practice-resources/state-advocacy/490-model-state-legislation. Accessed February 19, 2011.

7. Younger P, Conner C, Cartwright K, Kole S, Forsyth J. *Physician Assistant Legal Handbook: Aspen Law Center.* Gaithersburg, MD, Aspen Publishers; 1997, p. 80.

8. *Washington State Nurses Association v Board of Medical Examiners* 605P2d 1269 Wash. 1980.

9. AAPA Model Practice Act. 2009. Available at: http://www.aapa.org/advocacy-and-practice-resources/state-advocacy/490-model-state-legislation. Accessed February 19, 2011.

10. Younger P, Conner C, Cartwright K, Kole S, Forsyth J. *Physician Assistant Legal Handbook: Aspen Law Center.* Gaithersburg, MD, Aspen Publishers; 1997, p. 76.

11. Ibid.

Chapter 16

Common Sense Supervision

Supervision of physician assistants (PAs) can take many forms and have many variations. The adage applies here: "If you've seen one, you've seen one." The reason for variation is that each supervising physician and PA develop a relationship where supervision is mutually understood and is unique to the patient and provider needs.

Supervision is ultimately a function of shared expectations and trust. Setting expectations requires communication, dialogue, practice guidelines, and experience. Trust requires feedback to reinforce activities that are going well and to modify areas that need improvement. A well-functioning team with a PA needs to adapt to the changing needs of patients while, at the same time, adopting consistent practice guidelines and standard approaches to daily work.

The techniques of supervision can be thought of as occurring prospectively, concurrently, or retrospectively.[1]

Prospective supervision includes activities like writing the practice plan. A new PA graduate would be expected to present most or all of their cases concurrently, while an experienced PA might be expected to present a specific subset of patient cases, such as all cases sent to specialists or all complex cases. Agreeing to a practice plan and revisiting it at least once a year is a good approach to prospective supervision.

Concurrent supervision relies on an organized approach to the daily work of the medical team. Daily supervision is usually a combination of structured contact and unstructured contact. Structured contacts are activities like a morning huddle to review the patient lists for the day, or a lunchtime check-in. Unstructured contacts may be "curbside consults" in which the PA seeks the expertise of the supervising physician. In a new supervision relationship, the physician may specify a type of patient for which the PA always consults with the supervising physician.

Retrospective supervision is akin to quality control. The PA and the supervising physician should have a system for reviewing care already delivered. An effective method is for both the physician and the PA to pull old charts and to review the cases and outcomes together. These charts may include cases of specific diseases, procedures, types of care, random, or some other combination of criteria. (See **Table 16-1** for suggested retrospective review criteria.) A new working relationship benefits from more frequent and shorter retrospective review

Table 16–1 Types of Cases for Retrospective Review

Newer PA:
-All rx
-All antibiotics
-All narcotics
-All diabetics
-Random
Established PA with established supervisor:
-Unusual cases
-Procedure performed
-Random
Established PA with new supervisor:
-Complex case managed by PA
-Certain diagnoses
-Referral to specialist
-Referral to surgery
-Random

meetings, for example, weekly, biweekly, or monthly. Typical retrospective reviews for established PAs are done every 1 to 3 months.

Once the structure of supervision is established, the real work of supervision occurs in the interaction of presenting and discussing cases. Case discussions between a supervising physician and a PA are different from teaching rounds because the goal is mutual care of the patient, not training a medical student or resident who will practice independently in the future. The purpose of the presentation is to describe the patient as accurately as possible so that both providers can apply their skills and knowledge to the treatment of the case. A streamlined case presentation example is listed in **Table 16-2**.

Using positive and negative discriminating factors to create a differential diagnosis or a probable diagnosis allows both providers to match their "illness scripts."

> Expert clinicians store and recall knowledge as diseases, conditions, or syndromes — "illness scripts" —that are connected to problem representations. ... Constructed on the basis of exposure to patients, illness scripts are rich with clinically relevant information.[2]

Matching illness scripts with each other allows the physician to accurately assess the knowledge of the PA. A good match means they are seeing the case the same way. A poor match identifies a case that needs more investigation. A poor match might mean a lack of medical knowledge, a difference in prior experiences, or a difference in findings from the patient. With the differences highlighted, the team can revisit the differential of diagnostic possibilities and make an appropriate plan for the patient.

Table 16-2 Sample Illness Script

I have just seen patient _____who is _____years old with a chief complaint of _____for _____time. I believe his/her diagnosis is _____ because: List positive factors from history, physical exam, and diagnostic tests. And it is not _____: List other diseases considered in the differential diagnosis. Because_____: List negative findings which eliminate other diagnoses.

Source: Adapted from Bowen JL. Educational strategies to promote clinical diagnostic reasoning. *N Engl J Med.* 355;21:2217–2225.

Supervising and working with supervision is easy when there is no conflict. But conflict is inevitable in any relationship and will occur between physician and PA.[3] Conflict should be handled in a professional manner, with mutual respect and with the best interest of patients as the ultimate guide to resolution. Reviewing the structures used in PA supervision will help to resolve conflict. Revisiting the practice plan and the elements of prospective supervision can assist in identifying areas where structured supervision needs to be increased or relaxed. Evaluating the effectiveness of concurrent supervision might reveal that supervision activities are too time consuming or that they are not given enough time. A review of the preceding retrospective supervision meeting can identify new areas for retrospective review and can help determine whether reviews are too frequent or too far apart.

For the relationship to be successful, the supervising physician and the PA both need to get something positive out of the effort it takes to supervise and be supervised. For the physician, supervision might positively impact the physician's compensation or it might be a paid administrative function. Other non-monetary compensations for the supervising physician are listed in **Table 16-3**. The PA's reward is an excellent relationship with their supervising physician, allowing the PA to provide high-quality medical care within the medical team.

Table 16–3 Rewards of Supervising PAs

- Increased productivity of the team while there is decreased pressure on physician productivity.
- Decreased stress in patient care because there is a partner to discuss care and share the load.
- Increased flexibility for the physician to customize practice.
- Shorter days if the team can complete care more quickly than the physician alone in the past.
- Generalist physician's patients can benefit from a physician assistant with specialty experience.
- Specialized physician's patients can benefit from a physician assistant with primary care or general medicine experience.

Source: Data from AAPA 2009, National Physician Assistant Census Report. Available at: http://www.aapa.org/images/stories/Data_2009/National_Final_with_Graphics.pdf. Accessed January 8, 2011.

REFERENCES

1. Teherani A, O'Sullivan P, Aagaard E, Morrison EH, Irby DM. Student perceptions of the one minute preceptor and traditional preceptor models. *Medical Teacher*. 2007;29:323–327.
2. Bowen JL. Educational strategies to promote clinical diagnostic reasoning. *N Engl J Med*. 355;21:2217–2225.
3. Bing-You RG, Towbridge RL. Why medical educators may be failing at feedback. *JAMA*. 2009;302(12):1330–1331.

Chapter 17

Hospital Credentialing and Privileging

Newly practicing PAs are often surprised that their state license and national certifications are just the first steps to hospital practice. In addition, every hospital must also "credential" and "privilege" every healthcare practitioner working in the facility. These credentials and privileges must also be reviewed and updated periodically as part of an accreditation process for the hospital or healthcare delivery system.

The requirement for credentialing—which also applies to healthcare systems and some third-party payers—means that the healthcare provider must provide current information on training, certification, employment, malpractice status, and updated/required continuing medical education to the credentialing organization.

Individual facilities typically also require background checks, evidence of updated immunizations, and current Advanced Cardiac Life Support (ACLS) and Basic Cardiac Life Support (BCLS) certification. In addition, the credentialing organization checks with the National Practitioner Data Bank to assure that there are no actions—in any state—against the provider.

While providers working exclusively in the ambulatory portions of a delivery system generally required "credentialing" only, all providers participating in any component of hospital practice are required to be "privileged." Managed by the medical staff office—and involving some type of "peer review"—privileging requires the approval of specific activities for each provider. While there is generally an established list of typically approved procedures for each type of provider, the option to add additional specific procedures (often new technologies) on a case-by-case basis also exists.

Hospital privileges are established to meet the guidelines of the Joint Commission on the Accreditation of Healthcare Organizations (JCAHO or "The Joint Commission").

The Joint Commission (1997 Hospital Accreditation Standards) defines clinical privileges as authorization "to provide specific patient care services in the hospital within defined limits, based on the following factors, as applicable: license, education, training, experience, competence, health status and judgment."[1]

Providers go through a process—using institution-specific forms—to request privileges. For PAs, the supervising physician also signs those privilege requests. As in all other settings, the supervising physician is responsible for the practice of the PA. Patients admitted to the hospital are admitted to the physician's—or the practice's—service. A sample of hospital credentialing and privileging forms is available on the AAPA Web site (http://www.aapa.org/advocacy-and-practice-resources/practice-resources/hospital-practice/567). Privilege requests can often be very detailed; they delineate specific procedures. Providers may be required to provide detailed information—such as documentation of specific training or submission of patient logs—to verify their experience.

Once submitted, the credentialing and privileging requests are reviewed by the appropriate institutional committee in a "peer review" process. The intent is that an appropriate "peer" reviews the qualifications of each provider. Depending on the size and structure of the hospital, that peer might be someone of the same specialty.

In smaller hospitals peer review is not always possible. As the practice of PAs and NPs becomes more common in hospitals, the peer-review committee may include PAs and NPs to review those specific practitioners. Hospitals that have implemented this process have found this review to be very positive in providing a better understanding of the appropriate—and optimum—utilization of these providers.

When there are no PAs or NPs available on the review committee, PAs and NPs are most commonly reviewed and presented for approval by a physician from the service where the PA or NP is employed.

Periodic review of hospital privileges—required by The Joint Commission—are designed to review malpractice incidents, outcomes, and numbers of procedures performed to maintain competence. Privileges may be added or removed based upon this review.

All providers with approved hospital privileges are then governed by the by-laws, rules, regulations and policies, regardless of whether they are a member of the medical staff. The by-laws typically include a section on PA privileges, including the process for granting privileges.[2]

The American Academy of Physician Assistants (AAPA) has published *Guidelines for Amending Medical Staff Bylaws*.[3] This policy was most recently amended in 2003.

Key points of this document are quoted and or summarized below.

Definition of Physician Assistant　The physician assistant definition should be consistent with the AAPA's definition of a PA. This includes state licensure—unless the PA is employed by a federal entity, in which case federal rules apply.

> "Physician assistants (PAs)," according to the AAPA, "practice medicine with physician supervision. Typical hospital duties include evaluating and treating patients in the emergency room; performing histories and physicals; admitting patients on behalf of physicians; providing surgical first assisting for daily and emergency operating schedules; conducting patient rounds; evaluating changes in patients' conditions; issuing orders for medications, treatments and laboratory tests; and writing discharge summaries. PAs working with specialist physicians often have additional privileges particular to that field."[4]

Physician Assistants on the Medical Staff　Ideally PAs should be members of the medical staff—although there have been a number of misunderstandings about this issue. Medical staff attorneys may provide incomplete advice in this area in a misunderstanding of The Joint Commission's standards.

A critical issue is that PAs not be placed in the nursing category because they function under medical practice acts. Similarly, they should not be considered as Allied Health personnel—according to a number of policy documents on the National Commission on Allied Health which specifically exclude PAs and NPs from their definition.

Credentialing Physician Assistants   By-laws detail the criteria for credentialing each category of provider. Criteria spelled out by the Joint Commission include licensure details, training/experience, reference letters, and the ability to perform requested procedures.[5]

Physician Assistant Privileges

The privileges of PAs generally follow the template for physician privileges. According to the AAPA,

> The medical staff bylaws should stipulate that all clinical privileges granted to a physician assistant should be consistent with all applicable state and federal laws and regulations and that a physician assistant may provide medical and surgical services as delegated by a supervising physician.[2]

The criteria for granting privileges should be spelled out in the by-laws and is similar to those of the credentialing process.

Other Issues

Physicians and PAs are treated identically with regard to other issues in the by-laws including duration/renewal of clinical appointments, due process, quality assurance, corrective action, continuing education, committee appointments, and discrimination.

Participation in Disaster and Emergency Care   By-laws should be specific in enabling physician assistants to work in the system during emergency or disaster situations. This is particularly important because the designated supervising physician may not be readily available or accessible. Including physician assistants in the definition of providers authorized to provide care in these circumstances allows for maximum utilization of scarce personnel. The hospital emergency preparedness plan should be specific about the inclusion of physician assistants.[6]

CONCLUSION

Hospitals increasingly value the contribution that PAs make to their facilities. As PAs have become increasingly integrated into medical staffs, they have also begun to contribute to medical staff committees and other governance activities. Physician assistants and NPs frequently serve on credentialing and privileging committees and function as peer reviewers for their colleagues. Hospital privileges for PAs are better understood and facilitate quality care and improved outcomes.

REFERENCES

1. Joint Commission Standards and Resources. Available at: http://www .jcrinc.com/, page 125. Accessed March 30, 2010.
2. AAPA Issue Brief. *Physician Assistants in Hospital Practice: Credentialing and Privileging.* Available at: http://www.aapa.org/images/stories/IssueBriefs/ Hospital%20Practice/PAs%20in%20Hospital%20Practice%20-%202010 .pdf. Accessed November 10, 2010.
3. Hospital Credentialing and Privileging. Available at: http://www.aapa .org/advocacy-and-practice-resources/practice-resources/hospital- practice/567. Accessed on February 19, 2011.
4. American Academy of Physician Assistants, hospital practice: PAs in Hospital Practice: Credentialing and Privileging Jan 2010. Page 4, Available at: http://www.aapa.org/images/stories/hospitalc_p.pdf.
5. Younger P, Conner C, Cartwright K, Kole S, Forsyth J. *Physician Assistant Legal Handbook: Aspen Law Center.* Gaithersburg, MD: Aspen Publishers, Inc; 1997: 233.
6. AAPA Guidelines for Amending Hospital By-Laws. Available at: http:// www.aapa.org/advocacy-and-practice/hospital. Accessed March 30, 2010.

Chapter 18

Ethical Issues in Supervision

Garrett et al.[1] define a profession as members who are "dedicated to a particular life supportive of a particular expertise." They further define a profession as "a deep involvement in activities important to the functioning of society" and most importantly "a commitment to place service to society and often the individual ahead of, or at least equal to, personal gain." Physician assistants (PAs) are recognized by the profession, government, and patients as a profession and, as such, are expected to meet ethical and professional standards. Physicians, as members of the medical community and supervisors of PAs, have a responsibility to properly balance ethical principles with legal requirements and liabilities.[2]

While difficult to actually define, good ethics is a key component in proper supervision of a physician assistant. The traditional pyramid of health care with the physician at the top, responsible for all of the routine care of a patient, may not be as firm as it once was. According to Hooker et al., "The ideal relationship between a physician and a PA has not been fully articulated in spite of the rhetoric coming from the professional societies of physicians and PAs."[3] Byington believes that today's labyrinth of roles and responsibilities may create problems and concerns for the supervising physician–PA team, especially in terms of communication and decision-making.[4] In many settings, PAs have their own patient panels and greater independence seeking consultation. The assumption by some is that this means fewer interactions between PA and the supervising physician because PAs are capable of handling most patient care problems. Regardless of the validity of this statement, this is an appropriate time to reexamine the essential characteristics of a successful supervising physician–PA team.

Appropriate supervision is one of the central principles in the success of competent supervising physician–PA teamwork. Effective supervision means that the PA performs medical and/or surgical acts and procedures that have been authorized by state law and the supervising physician. The supervising physician bears both the authority and responsibility for the delegated acts. Obviously, methods of supervision vary with the practice setting, the comfort of the supervising physician, and the experience of the PA. It is common, early in the mentoring relationship, for supervision to be more formal and conservative and with experience to become less rigid as the team works together and rapport evolves.

The following four case studies address ethical issues in the relationship between supervising physician and physician assistant. These cases should encourage discussion between the supervising physician and the PA as they learn to work together as a team.

Case Study #1

During a routine examination performed by the PA, a patient requests a refill of a long-standing prescription for Vicodin® for chronic back pain. Since this is the first time he has seen the patient, the PA takes additional time to do a focused history and physical examination. He determines that there may be no indication to refill the narcotic. Because the patient has seen the supervising physician in the past, the PA consults with the supervising physician. While the PA is attempting to review the case with the supervising physician, the supervising physician, appearing very busy, abruptly says, "I know this patient—just give him the prescription." When the PA makes a second attempt to review the case with the physician, the supervising physician again interrupts and says, "Look, I'm the physician, just do what I say!"

Differences of opinion between the supervising physician and the PA are not particularly unhealthy nor should they be discouraged if they arise in an appropriate manner. It is also important to remember that, although supervision is a legal requirement, the PA still bears the ethical responsibility to ensure that patients receive proper and competent care. Case Study #1 clearly shows a problem in the relationship and communication between the supervising physician and the PA. It may be that the PA could have chosen a better time to interact with the supervising physician or the PA might have asked the supervising physician if the time was appropriate to speak about the case. On the other hand, the supervising physician should have enough respect for the PA to either take the time to interact constructively with the PA or to suggest a better time to speak. Conversely, the PA might have indicated to the supervising physician that he or she was uncomfortable with the direction given and might have asked the supervising physician to sign the order and then reschedule the patient with the supervising physician.

Case Study #2

A new graduate PA is hired by a physician in a solo practice. About a month into the relationship the physician approaches the PA and asks her to prescribe Percocet® for him for his chronic migraine headaches. He states he only takes it when his headaches are unbearable and does not want to leave the practice to be seen. The PA complies with the request. A week later the SP makes the same request to the PA, and once again the PA complies. A month later the physician is reported to the state medical board by a coworker regarding misuse of narcotics and potential impairment. The PA is also then referred to the PA board for inappropriate prescribing.

Reporting a supervising physician to the state regulatory board because of impairment, although an ethical requirement, is nonetheless difficult. This is even more complex when an employer–employee relationship is involved. Although this case deals with an impaired physician, the converse is also true. Both the supervising physician and the PA should have at the center of their efforts the safety and welfare of the patient. Supervising physicians and PAs should not be providers for each other. It is important to consult the state statutes and rules for more definition.

Case Study #3

The supervising physician finds out that the PA, who has been in the practice for over 3 years, has been treating an immediate family member for chronic urinary tract infections without completing and documenting an adequate history and physical examination. The supervising physician also finds out that the PA has been using medications from the office sample closet to treat the family member. This is brought to the supervising physician's attention when the primary care physician of the family member contacts the supervising physician to complain.

This case centers on boundary issues with family members, but could also pertain to friends and colleagues. First and foremost, PAs and supervising physicians should perform and appropriately document focused history and physical examinations on individuals where a legal physician–patient (or a PA–patient) relationship has occurred. Many state statutes consider treating an immediate family member as unethical conduct. As in previous cases, the relationship between the PA and SP is important. How sample medications should be utilized is a question that should be discussed early on in the supervising physician–PA relationship.

Case Study #4

The supervising physician confronts the PA when it becomes apparent, after talking with the patient, that the PA had listed a procedure (rectal examination) on the medical records, which actually had not been completed. The PA admits he had not actually done the examination and agrees to be more accurate in the future.

Dishonesty and improper charting is a serious offense. The supervising physician has to trust the PA and demand integrity. For the PA to admit the error is a positive sign. The supervising physician may want to increase the number of PA chart reviews as well as face-to-face meetings with the PA. There are multiple liability issues (e.g., billing fraud) with this case. Integrity should be a mainstay both for patient care and supervising physician–PA interactions.

Most physicians and PAs enjoy their professional relationship. The relationship between a PA and the supervising physician should be one of mutual trust and respect. The PA—first and foremost—is a representative of the physician, treating the patient in the style and manner developed and directed by the physician.

While there are no absolutes, the following eight characteristics were modified from an article in *Medscape Family Medicine*[5]; they are necessary for a successful and ethical supervising physician–PA team:

1. *Respect.* It is imperative for both the supervising physician–and the PA to have professional trust and respect for one another. This means supporting each other with patients, office staff, and colleagues. Disagreements or differences should be resolved in private. The PA is a representative or an extension of the physician, treating the patient in the style and manner developed and directed by the supervising physician This dependent relationship allows PAs to be utilized in multiple practice settings.

2. *Understanding of state statutes that govern supervision and PA practice.* First, the physician supervisor and the PA must know and understand rules and statutes that govern the PA's scope of practice and the supervision by the physician (see Appendix A). Secondly, the physician should be aware of guidelines for physician–PA practice from their professional organizations. **Table 18-1** shows the 1995 American Medical Association guidelines for physician–PA practice as approved by their House of Delegates.[6] Having a copy of the pertinent state statutes and rules that govern the practice of PAs is important and should be reviewed on an annual basis, just as it is important to review other standards, such as those from the Occupational Safety and Health Administration or standards for advanced life support.

Table 18–1 American Medical Association Suggested Guidelines for Physician-Physician Assistant Practice

Reflecting the comments from the American Academy of Physician Assistants, separate model guidelines for Physician/Physician Assistants practice have been developed. These are based on the unique relationship of physician assistants who recognize themselves as agents of physicians with respect to delegated medical acts, and legal responsibilities. They are consistent with the existing AMA policies concerning physician assistants cited in this report. The suggested guidelines reflect those as follows:

1. The physician is responsible for managing the health care of patients in all settings.
2. Healthcare services delivered by physicians and physician assistants must be within the scope of each practitioner's authorized practice, as defined by state law.
3. The physician is ultimately responsible for coordinating and managing the care of patients and, with the appropriate input of the physician assistant, ensuring the quality of health care provided to patients.
4. The physician is responsible for the supervision of the physician assistant in all settings.
5. The role of the physician assistant in the delivery of care should be defined through mutually agreed upon guidelines that are developed by the physician and the physician assistant and based on the physician's delegatory style.
6. The physician must be available for consultation with the physician assistant at all times, either in person or through telecommunication systems or other means.
7. The extent of the involvement by the physician assistant in the assessment and implementation of treatment will depend on the complexity and acuity of the patient's condition and the training, experience, and preparation of the physician assistant, as adjudged by the physician.
8. Patients should be made clearly aware at all times whether they are being cared for by a physician or a physician assistant.
9. The physician and physician assistant together should review all delegated patient services on a regular basis, as well as the mutually agreed upon guidelines for practice.

The physician is responsible for clarifying and familiarizing the physician assistant with his/her supervising methods and style of delegating patient care.

Source: Data from American Medical Association Suggested Guidelines for Physician-Physician Assistant Practice. Available at: http://aapa.org/advocacy-and-practice-resources/practice-resources/supervision/579. Accessed January 30, 2011.

3. *Understanding the PA's scope of practice.* This includes a description of the PA's role and responsibilities and a list of conditions that require immediate consultation with the supervising physician. Prospective discussion of expectations regarding patient care will assist in later problems or disagreements. The physician should be clear on what conditions, if any, require consultation before discharge. In many emergency centers, for example, standing orders require that consultation with the supervising physician regarding all chest pain or abdominal pain patients must occur before the patient leaves.

4. *Communication.* An "open door" policy or guidelines for accessibility to the supervising physician should be clearly established. It is important that the physician and PA avoid obstacles that impede access to discussions of patient care. The Pew Health Professions Commission in 1998 published the following recommendations for the traditional physician–PA team:

> The traditional relationship between PAs and physicians, the hallmarks of which are frequent consultation, referral, and review of PA practice by the supervising physician, is one of the strengths of the PA profession. The characteristics of this relationship are also considered to be the elements of professional relationships in any well-designed health system.[7]

5. *Recognition of each other's strengths.* The physician–PA team relationship can hinge on this factor. Early in the relationship the physician and PA should get to know each other's strengths and weaknesses. The delivered care should cater to the strengths of the PA and any weaknesses should be addressed with additional training or continuing medical education.

6. *Sharing clinical resources.* The physician–PA team should agree on clinical resources available in the practice setting. At a minimum the supervising physician–PA team should have access, either electronic or hardcopy, to various reference sources. In addition, appropriate equipment and diagnostic tools should be available, depending on the focus of the practice.

7. *Understanding the employer–employee relationship.* See Chapter 3 for more information on this relationship.

8. *Understanding legal billing requirements.* This is particularly important when it comes to Medicare. While Medicare requires compliance with state law, it also has its own requirements. Not complying with these requirements and billing for procedures not properly supervised may be grounds for charges of Medicare fraud. There are two types of supervision required under Medicare, "incident to" and "physician services." "Incident to" services are integral (although incidental) to a physician's professional service, commonly furnished in a physician's office. It requires a physician be present in the office (not particularly in the same room) and immediately available to the PA. Physician services, conversely, can be performed by PAs. These are broadly defined under Medicare as the services that are routinely performed by a physician. However, physician services performed by the PA that do not meet Medicare "incident to" criteria result in a reduced payment to the medical practice. The supervising physician–PA must understand these ramifications and must institute mutually understood practice standards.

A single chapter on ethical supervision cannot adequately cover the issues. A supervising physician and a PA must develop a sense of personal ethical integrity. Supervising PAs can be rewarding, cost-effective, and can enhance caring for patients. However, being ethical in that relationship by considering modern medical ethical issues and norms, by adhering to supervisory requirements, by avoiding tort liability through proper billing, and by creating a positive atmosphere for partnership will assist the physician and PA in meeting these goals.

REFERENCES

1. Garrett TM, Baillie HW, Garrett RM. *Health Care Ethics: Principles and Problems.* 4th ed. Boston, MA: Pearson Education, Prentice Hall; 2001: Ph 16.
2. Kao A. Ethics, law, and professionalism: What physicians need to know. In: Stern DT. *Measuring Medical Professionalism.* New York: Oxford University Press; 2006:39.

3. Hooker RS, Cawley JF, Asprey DP. *Physician Assistants: Policy and Practice.* 3rd ed. Philadelphia, PA: FA Davis; 2010:379.

4. Byington, M. The changing landscape of supervision. Forum: Supervision. Risk Management Foundation of the Harvard Medical Institutions; 1999. Available at: http://www/rmf.harvard.edu/publications/forum/v19n5/article1/body.html. Accessed February 12, 2002.

5. Danielsen RD. What factors are necessary for a successful PA/MD relationship? Medscape Family Medicine Web site. Available at: http://www.medscape.com/viewarticle/429407. Accessed January 10, 2010.

6. American Medical Association Web site. Health policies of AMA House of Delegates (HOD). AMA Advocacy Resource Center; 2006(update):8-9. Accessed January 6, 2010.

7. The Pew Health Professions Commission. Charting a Course for the Twenty-First Century: Physician Assistants and Managed Care. San Francisco, CA: UCSF Center for the Health Professions; 1998.

Chapter 19

Medical Liability and Physician Assistants

In addition to the longstanding issues of lack of patient access to health care and increasing cost, there are concerns about the safety and quality of care being delivered in the United States, especially as information on the nature and the extent of errors in health care and on medical malpractice have been brought to the forefront. In spite of extensive public education, the Agency for Healthcare Research and Quality (AHRQ) reported in 2007 that patient safety was improving at a disappointing 1% per year.[1] According to Sexton et al., the healthcare industry, dedicated to protecting lives, unfortunately has become the 8th leading cause of death.[2]

It has been rumored that PAs cannot be sued for malpractice. This is, of course, untrue. Since 1990, the National Practitioner Data Bank (NPDB) has been collecting information on healthcare practitioners, including PAs, with regard to disciplinary actions such as monetary judgments (both by settlement and jury decision), loss of licensure, and limitation of practice. Over the past 20 years, PAs have experienced increased liability, mostly as a result of their expanding scope of practice, greater patient care responsibilities, and increased autonomy. However, according to Crane's article in the March 2000 edition of

Medical Economics, "Judging from the actual number of malpractice cases settled, PAs and NPs are in court much less often than their doctor colleagues."[3]

Information from the NPDB, in fact, reveals that PAs incur a remarkably low rate of malpractice judgments. Moreover, anecdotal data support the possibility that hiring a PA may even reduce the risk of malpractice liability.[4]

The Health Care Quality Improvement Act, passed by Congress in 1986, requires that malpractice payments made on behalf of any clinician who is licensed, registered, or certified by the state must be reported to the NPDB.[5] Since the data bank began collecting statistics, it has recorded a total of 235,797 paid claims for physicians, with an average paid claim (inflation adjusted) of $282,782. During that same period, the NPDB recorded a total of 1130 paid claims for PAs, with an average paid claim of $86,568.[6] One can gain some perspective on these data by keeping in mind that, in 2006, there were 633,000 physicians, 125,000 NPs, and 70,000 PAs practicing in the United States. There were nine physicians for every PA at that time.

Notably, the number of physician-related paid claims approached 100 times that of PA-related paid claims. A further disparity was found when mean awards were compared: the 2006 mean physician-related awards were 1.33 times greater than PA-related awards ($312,000 for physicians versus $234,000 for PAs).[6] Unfortunately, the mean rate for PAs approached that of the physician.

Another way of examining the differences between the malpractice experiences of PAs and physicians is to calculate the applicable provider pool for each malpractice claim paid. Data from 2006 show that 1 claim was paid for every 50.6 physicians, compared to 1 for every 619.5 PAs.[6] (However, the accuracy of reports to the NPDB is unknown and variations exist from state to state, which may affect the reliability of the data.)

Each healthcare provider is responsible for his or her own negligent acts. Because a supervising physician is responsible for the actions of the PA, the PA is not exempt from the risk of individual liability. Malpractice is another word for "negligence," which means that a healthcare provider has not met the standard of care expected of reputable and careful healthcare providers under similar circumstances. If the malpractice caused harm, a lawsuit or claim can be filed to recover damages for the harm that was suffered.

To win a negligence case and recover damages from a PA, a patient (plaintiff) must prove 3 things: (1) that the PA owed the patient a *duty of care*, (2) that he or she *breached that duty*, and (3) that the patient was *harmed* as a result of the PA's action or failure to act. A PA's duty to a patient arises from the provider–patient relationship. That relationship exists when a PA has agreed to care for a patient. The scope of the PA's duty to a patient is called the standard of care. A PA who does not comply with the standard of care has breached the duty owed to the patient. If that breach causes harm to the patient, the PA may be found negligent. The standard of care is determined, usually, by testimony of other PAs, known as expert witnesses, establishing what a reasonable and prudent PA would do in the reported circumstances.[7] When a PA has, or professes to have, a particular expertise, the standard of care may be higher.

Conduct that may lead to liability includes failure to properly diagnose, failure to refer, exceeding one's scope of practice, negligent monitoring, failure to question a physician's abnormal order, or failure to properly follow-up.

A patient seeking damages from a PA must prove that the PA's breach of duty caused the patient to suffer harm. In legal terms, the plaintiff (patient) must prove that the PA's error was the proximate cause of the injury. Proximate causes have been described as a foreseeable, natural, or direct cause.

What should the PA expect when a lawsuit is filed? Once a lawsuit has been filed with the Court,

1. The plaintiff (patient) serves the PA with a summons
2. Prelitigation activity takes place (which may take months)
3. The complaint is formally reported
4. The PA meets with his or her defense attorney
5. Preanswer motions are filed (which may take more months)
6. Discovery occurs (e.g., asking for particular materials, records, etc.)

7. Interrogatories take place (i.e., questions between plaintiff and defense attorneys)
8. Depositions occur with the defendant PA and any and all expert witnesses
9. Trial alternatives are discussed (in some states pretrial screening panels are required)
10. Abitration may be required or may take place
11. Settlement or trial takes place

In most cases, PAs are covered under their employer's malpractice insurance policy. Nevertheless, they may still be held liable for negligence and may still be liable for all or part of a plaintiff's award or settlement. It is important, in the author's opinion, that PAs maintain their own personal medical liability insurance (**Table 19-1**). The PA's first action when learning of a claim should be to contact the malpractice carrier. Failing to do so may violate the policy of the malpractice carrier and result in denial of coverage.

An exception is made for PAs and physicians who work within the federal government (i.e., in the military, in public health service, or in federal facilities). For these individuals, the Federal Tort Claims Act (FTCA) provides a limited waiver of the federal government's sovereign immunity when its employees are negligent within the scope of their employment. Under the FTCA, the government can only be sued

Table 19-1 Malpractice Insurance Carriers for Physician Assistants

Name	Web Address	Phone
American Academy of Physician Assistants	www.epreceptor.com/aapa_insurance/index.html	877-356-2272
CM&F Group	www.cmfgroup.com/Insurance_products/professional_liability_individual/physician_assistant.html	800-221-4904
Healthcare Providers Service Organization	www.hpso.com/professional-liability-insurance/physician-assistant-coverage.jsp	888-273-4686

under circumstances in which the United States, if a private person, would be liable to the claimant in accordance with the law of the place where the act or omission occurred. Therefore, the FTCA does not apply to conduct that is uniquely governmental (e.g., incapable of performance by a private individual).[8]

Multiple articles and handbooks discuss methods of avoiding medical liability, such as the *Physician Assistant Legal Handbook*[7] by Aspen Health Law and Compliance Center. They all make the following basic recommendations:

1. Know and understand your scope of practice under state law
2. Know and understand your hospital or institutional policies
3. Know and understand the importance of communicating honestly with your patients and your supervising or collaborating physician
4. Know and understand the importance of communication between the PA and the supervising physician
5. Document, document, and document

Ensuring patient safety and improving quality of care are steadfast goals for all PAs and their supervising physicians.

REFERENCES

1. US Department of Health and Human Services, Agency for Healthcare Research and Quality. *National Healthcare Quality Report 2007*. Rockville, MD: US Department of Health and Human Services; 2008.
2. Sexton JB, Thomas EJ, Helmreich RL. Error, stress and teamwork in medicine and aviation: Cross sectional surveys. *BMJ*. 2000;320: 745–749.
3. Crane M. NPs and PAs: What's the malpractice risk? *Med Econ*. 2000; 77:205–208.
4. Levinson W, Roter DL, Mullooly JP, et al. Physician–patient communication: The relationship with malpractice claims among primary care physicians and surgeons. *JAMA*. 1997;277(7):553–559.
5. National Practitioner Data Bank Web site. Health Care Quality Improvement Act. Available at: http://www.npdb-hipdb.hrsa.gov/legislation/title4.html. Accessed March 12, 2010.

6. US Department of Health and Human Services. The National Practitioner Data Bank Research File. Maintained by the Division of Quality Assurance, Bureau of Health Professions, Health Resources and Services Administration. Available at: http://www.npdb-hipdb.hrsa .gov/. Accessed June 10, 2010.

7. Younger P, Conner C, Cartwright K, Kole S, Forsyth J. *Physician Assistant Legal Handbook: Aspen Law Center.* Gaithersburg, MD: Aspen Publishers, Inc; 1997:63.

8. 'Lectric Law Library Web site. Available at: http://www.lectlaw.com/def/ f071.htm. Accessed March 12, 2010.

Specific Practice Settings

Chapter 20

Ambulatory Care and Emergency Medicine

The delivery of health care in the United States is a complex process. It occurs in hospitals and outpatient settings—the offices of primary care providers and specialists—urgent care centers and emergency departments. What differentiates primary care and ambulatory care? What impacts have patient preference, advancements in technology, and health insurance had on the delivery of medical care? What are the contributions of emergency medicine and urgent care? The answers to these questions are based on an appreciation of the past, reflections on the present and projections into the future.

In the simplest terms, the practice of medicine can be viewed as being composed of two interacting variables: (1) the *type* of care provided and (2) the *location* where that care is delivered. There are two types of care (primary care and specialty care) and two locations for the delivery of care (inpatient care and ambulatory care). The term "primary care" gained status in the United States in 1961.[1] It has been described as consisting of four fundamental features: (1) the patient's access to the health care system through a first-point of contact, (2) a longitudinal nature of care (i.e., continuous), (3) comprehensive scope, and (4) integration of all elements of the patient's care (i.e., coordinated).[2] Specialty care is generally delivered in 1 of 2 manners:

consultative or ongoing. In a consultative situation, patients are referred to a specialist who assists in establishing an uncertain diagnosis by performing diagnostic or therapeutic procedures and/or providing recommendations for treatment. Some diagnoses are so infrequent or complex that they require the expertise of a specialist for an extended (ongoing) period of time.

Ambulatory care is not synonymous with primary care. While primary care is defined by the nature of the care provided, ambulatory care is characterized by the location where the care is delivered. Ambulatory care is essentially all healthcare delivered to patients who are not confined to an institutional setting (i.e., a hospital ward, inpatient status). Based on, but not limited to, advances in technology, patients' desire for convenience, and attempts to reduce the costs of healthcare delivery, the past few decades have witnessed a shift from inpatient to outpatient care. In 2006, almost 80% of ambulatory care was delivered in physicians' offices, more than 50% by primary care providers (e.g., general and family medicine 23.1%, internal medicine 13.9%, and pediatrics 13.6%).[3] Therefore, a large percentage of ambulatory care is provided by specialists, the most common reason being routine or preventative care for nonreferred patients.[4] If more services were provided by primary care providers, patient care might be better coordinated. Various healthcare delivery plans, the most recent being the "patient-centered medical home" (PCMH) have been designed to reform healthcare delivery in this direction.

Health insurance plans (especially those referred to as managed care) were primarily designed to improve the quality of care and/or to reduce the cost of healthcare delivery. Managed care is an attempt to organize providers, methods of payment, and insurers to accomplish these goals. Although a number of permutations of managed care models exist, historically the three most common are these: (1) health maintenance organizations (HMOs), (2) preferred provider organization (PPOs), and (3) point-of-service (POS) plans. In the simplest terms, managed care can be viewed as being composed of two interacting features: (1) access to health care (i.e., the presence or absence of a gatekeeper, the contact person who authorizes or denies requested services) and (2) provision of health care through an organized network of providers, often specialists.[5] HMOs have both a gatekeeper and network. PPOs provide care through a network but do not have a gatekeeper. POS plans have a gatekeeper but not a network. During the 17 years from 1998 to 2005, the percentage of employer-provided healthcare insurance delivered through a managed care plan increased from 27% to 97%; healthcare costs also continued to accelerate.[5] The PCMH concept is touted to be capable of providing improved patient outcomes with reduced costs through a team-based, technologically enhanced model of care. Recent estimates project that, if every patient had a primary-care physician (rather than various specialists) providing the majority of their medical needs through a PCMH, the United States would save $67 billion per year on healthcare costs.[6] If the United States continues to move toward this type of healthcare reform, the need for primary-care providers and the number of ambulatory care visits will both increase.

At the crossroads of primary care and specialty care, inpatient and ambulatory settings, resides emergency care. Although intended for unanticipated, acute, or severe illnesses or injury, emergency care is increasingly the point of first contact for non-emergent medical care. As the care delivered in emergency departments and urgent care centers is neither continuous nor comprehensive, better coordination through the office of primary-care providers must once again be considered.

Since 1974, data from the American Academy of Physician Assistants (AAPA) and the National Commission on the Certification of Physician Assistants (NCCPA) show notable changes in the practices of PAs; there has been a reduction from 69.8% to 34.2% in primary care with an increase from 1.3% to 12.4% in emergency medicine.[7,8] As PAs practice with physicians, it is not surprising that this pattern parallels that of the physician workforce. Recent trends in the specialty choice of graduating medical students as well as career changes among practicing physicians are driven by income potential and work hours, and they appear to be heavily dependent (between 37% and 55% of variability) upon controllable lifestyle (i.e., time for avocational pursuits and family activities).[9] The literature specific to PA students and PAs is not as robust or recent; however, the variables appear to share certain commonalities.[10] The increasing numbers of PAs and their expanding scope of practice, the public's enhanced awareness of the PA profession, and growing employment opportunities through physician practices and managed care organizations continue to broaden lifestyle options as well as geographic opportunities.

Adding to the milieu of increasing healthcare costs and shifts in the healthcare workforce to more specialists, by 2016 the number of individuals in the United States who are 55 years of age or older is projected to increase from 67 million (i.e., 29.3% of the population in 2006) to 87 million (i.e., 34.8% of the population).[11] As this group has been shown to experience increasing morbidity and to require more medical care, healthcare delivery needs, especially for the number of primary care providers, are expected to grow comparably.

The basic reality of any forecasting model is that, at best, it provides an educated guess. The output of any forecasting model is based upon its input, usually a combination of historical data and expert opinion. Attempting to devise a formula or template upon which to design training programs that will increase the production of primary care providers is no different. With those qualifiers, what can training programs do to help shape the future?

The most important predictors of the likelihood that a student will enter a primary care field upon graduation are the characteristics and preferences that a student brings with him or her into the program.[12] Let me repeat that: The measurable attributes that a student already possesses when entering a training program are the most important determinants of a career in primary care. Experiences during the clerkship phase of training can support and further develop the student's interest; they usually do not create the interest.[12] If a program truly wants to increase its output of graduates who will choose primary care as a career, then it must develop and refine an admissions process that increases the intake of students with characteristics, congruent with legal parameters, that have been reported to predispose them to this choice. Characteristics that have been reported in various studies to be associated with a greater likelihood of entering primary care include the following:

1. Expecting a lower income
2. Being married
3. Being female
4. Being older (nontraditional) at matriculation
5. Having parents who are not physicians
6. Having parents with a lower income
7. Being able to use a breadth of knowledge in one's practice
8. Being interested in the delivery of longitudinal care.[13,14]

In conclusion, the delivery of medical care services in an ambulatory setting will continue to increase. The need for primary care providers will increase over the next 10 years and beyond. Discussions are currently underway that may be swinging the pendulum back toward the production of more primary care providers than specialists. It appears that the most effective mechanism to produce clinicians that will enter a career in primary care is to recruit and accept into training programs students who already possess characteristics that align them with that destiny.

REFERENCES

1. White KL, Williams TF, Greenberg BG. The ecology of medical care. N Engl J Med. 1961;265:885–893.
2. Starfield B. *Primary Care: Balancing Health Needs, Services and Technology.* New York, NY: Oxford University Press; 1998.
3. Cherry DK, Hing E, Woodwell DA, Rechtsteiner EA. National Ambulatory Medical Care Survey: 2006 Summary. *National Health Statistics Reports.* 2008;3:1–40.
4. Valderas JM, Starfield B, Forrest CB, et al. Ambulatory care provided by office-based specialists in the United States. *Ann Fam Med.* 2009;7:104–111.
5. Folland S, Goodman AC, Stano M. *The Economics of Health and Health Care.* 5th ed. Boston, MA: Pearson; 2007.

6. Arnst C. The family doctor: A remedy for health-care costs? *Businessweek.* 2009(Jul 6):34–37.

7. Cawley JF. Physician assistants and Title VII support. *Acad Med.* 2008;83:1049–1056.

8. Arbet SA, Lathrop J, Hooker RS. Using practice analysis to improve the certifying examinations for PAs. *JAAPA.* 2009;22:31–36.

9. Dorsey ER, Jarjoura D, Rutecki GW. Influence of controllable lifestyle on recent trends in specialty choice by US medical students. *JAMA.* 2003;290:1173–1178.

10. Singer AM, Hooker PA. Determinants of specialty choice of physician assistants. *Acad Med.* 1996;71:917–919.

11. Dohm A, Shipner L. Occupational employment projections to 2016. *Month Labor Rev.* 2007;11:86–105.

12. Gazewood JD, Owen J, Rollins LK. Effect of generalist preceptor specialty in a third-year clerkship on career choice. *Fam Med.* 2002;34: 673–677.

13. Senf JH, Campos-Outcalt D, Kutob R. Factors related to the choice of family medicine. *J Am Board Fam Practice.* 2003;16:502–512.

14. DeWitt DE, Curtis JR, Burke W. What influences career choices among graduates of a primary care training program? *J Gen Int Med.* 1998;13:257–261.

Chapter 21

Hospital-Based Practice

Commonly, in the past century, primary care physicians were intimately involved in the admission, care, and discharge of their hospitalized patients. In fact, this took up a great deal of their preclinic, lunchtime, and postclinic hours during both weekdays and weekends. In large cities this may have taken up a great deal of travel time in a busy physician's day.[1] Once the PA became a common extension of the physician's practice, PAs were also asked to take on many of the hospital tasks for their patients.

Sometime in the late 1990s, this all changed with the advent of hospital-based practice. To alleviate the burden of the office-based physician, hospitalists were physicians whose main practice was within the walls of the hospitals, or in some cases multiple hospitals. These physicians cared for patients admitted through the emergency center or outpatient clinics. In 1996 Wachter used the term "hospitalist" in the *New England Journal of Medicine*.[2] Shortly thereafter, the National Association of Inpatient Physicians (NAIP) was born. In 2003 the NAIP changed its name to the Society of Hospital Medicine (SHM). At this writing, the SHM is the only medical organization dedicated, entirely to hospitalists.[3] The SHM publishes *The Journal of Hospital Medicine*, the only peer-reviewed journal for hospital medicine.

As one of the fastest-growing specialties in the United States, it is not surprising that PAs are starting to play a larger role in this practice. More than 400 PAs currently work as hospitalists, compared to more than 28,000 physicians.[1]

According to Hooker, PAs in hospitals "can prescribe narcotics, undertake procedures, and direct patient care with fewer restrictions than in outpatient settings."[4] In some instances, Hooker contends, PAs may serve as inpatient specialists relieving the work of the physician. It is reasonable to think that having a PA on the hospitalist's team will free up physicians to spend more time with patients in a cost-effective manner.

The very nature of hospitalist medicine, combined with the generalist nature of PAs, makes this field appealing to both physicians and PAs. The flexibility of the practice as well as the ability to choose between general and specialty work has encouraged more PAs to consider hospital-based practice.

While all PA educational programs prepare the PA for a generalist credential, considered a mainstay of the profession, this also becomes one of the biggest challenges when a PA wants to move into a hospitalist practice. A PA who wants to work in hospital medicine needs to acquire additional skills, including the ability to interact with a large array of hospital team members. **Table 21-1** contains the policy of the Society of Hospital Medicine regarding the utilization of PAs.

Table 21-1 SHM Policy Statements on Physician Assistants and Nurse Practitioners in Hospital Medicine[5]

SHM acknowledges the expanding role of Physician Assistants and Nurse Practitioners in hospital medicine and supports their continued integration in a collaborative healthcare system given the following guidelines:

1. The hospitalist is responsible for supervising Physician Assistants and/or Nurse Practitioners sharing in the care of the hospitalist's patients.[a]

2. Health care services delivered by Physician Assistants and/or Nurse Practitioners must be within the scope of the hospitalist physicians' or designee's authorized practice, as defined by state law, the medical practice act, and the credentialing hospital(s).[b]

3. The hospitalist must be available for consultation with the Physician Assistant and/or Nurse Practitioner at all times, either in person or through telecommunication systems or other means.[c]

4. The extent of the involvement by Physician Assistants and/or Nurse Practitioners in the assessment and implementation of treatment will depend on the complexity and acuity of the patient's condition and the training, experience, and preparation of the Physician Assistant and/or Nurse Practitioner as determined by the hospitalist physician or designee.[d]

5. SHM endorses the principle that the appropriate ratio of Physician Assistants and/or Nurse Practitioners should be determined by hospitalists at the practice level, consistent with good medical practice and state law where relevant.[e]

6. SHM supports Hospital bylaws that allow for the integration of Physician Assistants and Nurse Practitioners into hospitalist practices.

7. SHM supports the inclusion of Physician Assistants and/or Nurse Practitioners as part of a hospital medical staff.

8. Patients should be made aware at all times whether they are being cared for by a Physician Assistant and/or Nurse Practitioner in affiliation with a hospitalist.[f]

The above statements have been adapted from position statements from The American College of Physicians and the American Medical Association.

Note a: AMA H-35.989 Physician's Assistants, H-35.996 Status and Utilization of New or Expanding Health Professionals in Hospitals, H-160.947 Physician Assistants and Nurse Practitioners, H- 160.950 Guidelines for Integrated Practice of Physician and Nurse Practitioner, and ACP Expanding Roles of Nurse Practitioners and Physician Assistants Position Paper January 22, 2000 Position 1, Position 4.

Note b: AMA H-35.989 Physician's Assistants, H-35.996 Status and Utilization of New or Expanding Health Professionals in Hospitals, H-160.947 Physician Assistants and Nurse Practitioners, and H- 160.950 Guidelines for Integrated Practice of Physician and Nurse Practitioner.

Note c: AMA H-35.989 Physician's Assistants, H-160.947 Physician Assistants and Nurse Practitioners, and H-160.950 Guidelines for Integrated Practice of Physician and Nurse Practitioner.

Note d: AMA H-35.996 Status and Utilization of New or Expanding Health Professionals in Hospitals, H- 160.947 Physician Assistants and Nurse Practitioners, and H-160.950 Guidelines for Integrated Practice of Physician and Nurse Practitioner.

Note e: AMA H-35.975 Ratio of Physician to Physician Extenders.

Note f: AMA H-160.947 Physician Assistants and Nurse Practitioners and H-160.950 Guidelines for Integrated Practice of Physician and Nurse Practitioner.

Approved by SHM Board October 15, 2004

Source: Society of Hospital Medicine Policy Statements on Physician Assistants and Nurse Practitioners in Hospital Medicine. The Society of Hospital Medicine Web site available at: http://www.hospitalmedicine .org/AM/Template.cfm?Section=Practice_Resources&Template=/CM/ HTMLDisplay.cfm&ContentID=16738. Accessed January 5, 2010.

The SHM also publishes position-specific competencies for PAs working as hospitalists. Those competencies are shown in **Table 21-2**.

Miller et al.[6] suggest that the PA hired as a hospitalist may have three distinct roles, depending on the practice setting. The first is that of a first responder to patients requiring admission. The PA in this role acquires a history and performs a physical examination and creates a treatment plan either in the emergency department or

Table 21–2 PA Hospitalist Position Specific Competencies[5]

In addition to the following essential competencies, other competencies may be required to meet changing organization needs.

1. **Uses an appropriate problem-solving approach to plan services.**
   a. Performs complete medical history and physical exam on patients. Establishes differential diagnosis.
   b. Orders appropriate lab and diagnostic procedures.
   c. Synthesizes data to determine primary diagnosis and therapeutic plan utilizing established medical principles.
   d. Demonstrates the ability to recognize and critically assess any changes in patient's condition and reports such to the hospitalist physician.
   e. Coordinates acquisition of outpatient records from primary care provider or referring provider.
   f. Acts as a liaison and facilitator between hospitalist, staff members, case managers, and attending physician regarding patients.
   g. Rounds with and without hospitalist attending ensuring all lab work, diagnostic results, and other test results are available on chart and notifies hospitalist as appropriate.
   h. Facilitates coordination and development of a comprehensive and individual plan of care in collaboration with patient, family, and multidisciplinary team.
   i. Acts as a hospitalist service liaison with patient care staff.
   j. Facilitates one on one communication with primary care physician regarding current and ongoing patient care needs.
2. **Provides services with consideration of recipients needs.**
   a. Interprets and integrates patient data to determine appropriate diagnostic and therapeutic procedures needed.
   b. Prepares written prescription orders, medications, and controlled substances under the rules and regulations of the State of North Carolina and Federal DEA.

    c. Applies approved criteria to monitor appropriateness of hospital admissions and continued stays.

    d. Monitors implementation of guidelines for appropriateness of resources, trends and tracks guideline variances.

    e. Triages patient/family calls after discharge and up to first outpatient follow-up visit.

    f. Provides follow up with patient/family after discharge in conjunction with team member activity.

    g. Identifies appropriate venue for care within the continuum.

3. Uses equipment and supplies.

    a. Follows established procedures for computer and PDA.

    b. Follows manufacturer's guidelines for all equipment usage.

4. Uses appropriate safety and infection control measures.

    a. Corrects situations that pose a threat to patient or staff safety.

    b. Maintains BSI precautions.

5. Teaches/directs/advises/informs others in an appropriate manner.

    a. Participates in MD TRU Rounds.

    b. Ensures and maintains consensus related to entire hospital course from patient, family, physician, and payer.

    c. Coordinates patient and family education with nursing staff, ancillary staff, and other resources.

    d. Communicates with patients/families to ensure understanding of discharge instructions.

    e. Formulates, implements, and evaluates strategies for specialized education as it relates to patient care.

    f. Utilizes critical thinking and problem solving techniques.

    g. Is able to work independently, exercising sound judgment, discretion, and initiative to facilitate change.

6. Reports/records information appropriately.

    a. Dictates patient information in appropriate format and following established guidelines.

    b. Maintains daily progress notes using established guidelines.

    c. Follows all established HIMS policies for maintenance and signing of medical records.

Source: Society of Hospital Medicine Policy Statements on Physician Assistants and Nurse Practitioners in Hospital Medicine. The Society of Hospital Medicine Web site available at: http://www.hospitalmedicine .org/AM/Template.cfm?Section=Practice_Resources&Template=/CM/ HTMLDisplay.cfm&ContentID=16738. Accessed January 5, 2010.

after directly admitting the patient. The PA, in this role, may also be involved with rapid response, and may be a member of the Code Blue team. The second role is that of a unit-based provider. The PA in this role provides direct patient care along with a supervising hospitalist physician and may staff a single unit within the hospital. The third role may be that of a traditional hospitalist providing many of the tasks noted in Table 21-1.

The use of PAs in partnership with hospitalist physicians can and should enhance the quality of care for hospitalized patients. Creating continuity of care with a positive rapport with patients and families, PAs are important members of the hospitalist healthcare team.

REFERENCES

1. Hoppel A. Hospitalists: Ensuring quality care. *Clinician Reviews.* 2009;19(8):1.
2. Wachter R. The emerging role of hospitals in the emerging healthcare system. *N Eng J Med.* 1996;335(7):514–517.
3. Society of Hospital Medicine Web site. Available at: http://www .hospitalmedicine.org/Content/NavigationMenu/AboutSHM/ GeneralInformation/General_Information.htm. Accessed January 4, 2010.
4. Hooker RS. Physician assistants and nurse practitioners: The United States experience. *Med J Australia.* 2006;185(1):4.
5. The Society of Hospital Medicine Web site. Policy statements on physician assistants and nurse practitioners in hospital medicine. Available at: http://www.hospitalmedicine.org/AM/Template .cfm?Section=Practice_Resources&Template=/CM/HTMLDisplay .cfm&ContentID=16738. Accessed January 5, 2010.
6. Miller JA, Nelson J, Whitcomb W. Use of nonphysician clinical staff in hospitalist programs. In: Miller JA, Nelson J, Winthrop F, Whitcomb W. *Hospitalists: A Guide to Building and Sustaining a Successful Program.* Chicago, IL: Health Administration Press; 2007:101–110.

Chapter *22*

Assisted Living/Nursing Home Practice

The well-known medical and societal needs of the population aged 65 and over in the United States remain unmet. Unfortunately only a small number of clinicians in this country appear to be engaged in the care of assisted-living or nursing home patients. According to the Institute of Medicine, only 7100 geriatricians (and that number is declining), 1600 geriatric psychiatrists, less than 1% of nurses and pharmacists, and less than 4% of social workers specialize in geriatrics.[1] Over the past 20 years, attention has focused on the utilization of physician assistants (PAs) to extend and compliment the medical care in these practice settings.[1] As far back as 1988, Bottom introduced the PA and reported on trends that indicated that PAs were prepared to help fill the gaps in the health care of the elderly.[2] Although only 1% (approximately 7700) of PAs have chosen geriatrics as their practice, that number appears to be rising.[1] Because of the constant transportation problems with patients in assisted living and nursing facilities, utilization of on-site care by PAs eliminates that problem. The generalist training of PAs make them valuable clinicians in assisted living and nursing facility settings.

PAs may be employed by group practices, health maintenance organizations (HMOs), participating physicians, or other third-party payers. According to Caprio,[3] more than 20% of nursing facilities reported the use of PAs (and NPs). Physician assistants provide a wide array of services such as subacute and urgent care, preventive care, end-of-life care, and wound care. A 1998 study by Ackerman and Kemle revealed that the utilization of PAs in nursing homes reduced the number of hospital admissions by 38%.[4]

In addition, Hooker et al. report that PAs

> can provide the therapy team (which may include a physical therapist, an occupational therapist, a physiatrist, a rehabilitation nurse, and a psychologist) with an overview of the patient's chronic and acute medical problems, level of disability, level of cognitive impairment, drug history (including current therapy), and other factors that may impact formulation or progress of a rehabilitation program.[5]

Potential cost savings from the utilization of PAs have been reported in multiple studies over the years. The Centers for Medicare and Medicaid services established regulations regarding the utilization of PAs in skilled-nursing facilities. Physician assistants may perform medically necessary services within their scope as defined by state law. Although PAs in most settings perform comprehensive exams and assessments, only physicians may perform the full comprehensive visit in skilled nursing facilities (SNFs), but physicians may delegate follow-up visits as medically necessary.

As the need for onsite medical care increases, as more facilities embrace a medical model of care, and as the baby boomers seek this type of care, more collaboration between PAs and their supervising physicians will occur. As Brugna et al. reported in *Clinical Geriatrics*, "Physician assistants are well positioned to contribute to caring for our elderly population," and "a PA can assume the role of a geriatric assessment with a focus on the functional status, cognitive status, and special needs of the patient."[6]

Currently there are no postgraduate programs in geriatrics for the PA. The Society of Physician Assistants Caring for the Elderly (SPACE) is a fairly new focus group of the American Academy of Physician Assistants (AAPA) dedicated to gathering and disseminating information about PAs practicing in geriatric medicine. Their

Web site (http://www.geri-pa.org/) answers questions and provides links to related issues, suggests experienced speakers, provides a listing of training programs and helps to facilitate liaisons with other organizations who work with elderly patients.[7]

REFERENCES

1. Institute of Medicine of the National Academies. Retooling for an aging America—Building the healthcare workforce. April 11, 2008. Consensus Report.
2. Bottom WD. Geriatric medicine in the United States: New roles for physician assistants. *J Comm Health*. 1988;13(2):95–103.
3. Caprio TV. Physician practice in the nursing home: Collaboration with nurse practitioners and physician assistants. *Annals of Long Term Care*. 2006;14:17–24.
4. Ackerman RJ, Kemle KA. The effect of a physician assistant on the hospitalization of nursing home residents. *J Am Geriatr Soc*. 1998;46(5):610–614.
5. Hooker RK, Cawley JF, Asprey DP. *Physician assistants: Policy and Practice*. 3rd ed. Philadelphia, PA: FA Davis; 2010, p. 234.
6. Brugna RA, Cawley JF, Baker MD. Physician assistants in geriatric medicine. *Clin Geriatr*. 2007;15(10);NPN.
7. Society of Physician Assistants Caring for the Elderly (SPACE) Web site. Available at: http://www.geri-pa.org/Home/about-space. Accessed January 2, 2010.

Chapter 23

Geographically Remote Practice Site

Acknowledging the important role that PAs perform in access to health care, all 50 states provide for some sort of remote site practice.[1] The regulations around remote site practice—sometimes called "satellite practice"—vary greatly from state to state.

Each physician–PA team must be aware of their state's specific definitions and regulations for PA practice in remote sites. Because state practice acts are revised regularly, the individual state licensing body should be consulted. The American Academy of Physician Assistants (AAPA) maintains up-to-date information on PA practice in a state-by-state format in their document "Summary of State Laws for Physician Assistants."[2] That document is the primary source for the specific materials in this chapter.

In addition to information about specific state laws, the AAPA has created "Model State Legislation for Physician Assistants"[3] as a resource for states that are upgrading laws and regulations or even for the national licensing process. The model law specifically supports remote site practice, stating:

> Nothing contained herein shall be construed to prohibit the rendering of services by a physician assistant in a setting geographically remote from the supervising physician.[3]

Many state laws have "generic" rules about remote site practice; they simply state that the physician is not required to be on-site for PA practice as long as they are readily available for supervision by phone or electronic communication. Other states have detailed rules defining remote site practice and delineating the amount of time the physician must spend in the practice, setting specific requirements for chart review, and creating other requirements for the physician–PA team. Many states require that the PA receive specific permission for remote site practice through a process that includes a needs assessment and a specific supervision plan, including a plan for alternate supervision in the absence of the physician.

Ten states explicitly require "board approval" of remote site practice settings (see **Figure 23-1**).

Overall, remote site practice rules and regulations are seen as supportive of healthcare access but are seen as opposing practice arrangements that give any perception or impression of PA independence or autonomy. Some states require that remote sites have signage that

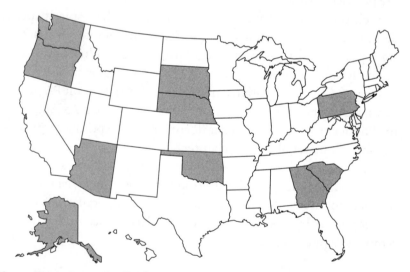

Figure 23–1 States Explicitly Requiring "Board Approval" of Remote Site Practice Settings. © Dr_Flash/ShutterStock, Inc.

clearly indicates the PA status of the clinician as well the supervision of the designated specific supervising physician.

Remote sites are often created to assure that primary-care clinics remain open in small communities even when hospitals are no longer viable. Generally linked to larger healthcare delivery systems such as regional hospitals or systems of community health centers, remote sites can be used to stabilize frail healthcare systems in rural communities. Remote site practice may also be used as a strategy to provide specialty consultation and follow-up in areas geographically removed from larger hospital centers. In some states, the remote-site practice definition applies to rotating medical coverage in nursing homes, correctional facilities, and other institutional settings.

Typically, the most rural states have the most liberal definitions of what constitutes a remote site. In Alaska, for example, PAs may practice in remote Aleutian Island settings with only electronic communication back to physicians in Anchorage—many hundreds of miles away.[1] Other licensing boards in more populated states may restrict remote sites according to the distance from the supervising physician's regular practice. For example, Delaware requires that supervising physicians be within a 30-minute distance. The state of Ohio says that the physician must be within a 60-minute travel time to the PA's location.[1] Other states, such as Missouri, limit PA practice to locations where the physician is no further than 30 miles away. South Carolina uses both mileage (45 miles) and travel time (60 minutes) to define remote site practices. Indiana requires that the physician and the PA be in the same or adjacent counties. Three states—Colorado, Georgia, and Texas—limit remote site practice to clinics serving the underserved or in governmentally designated areas with a shortage of health professionals, as a strategy to prevent PAs from establishing what might be lucrative independent practices.[2]

Six states are specific about the experience of the PA seeking to work in a remote practice. The issue of who should be eligible for remote site practice has historically been a controversial issue. (Most PA educators do not feel that new graduates should be hired for remote practice settings.) While some states explicitly prohibit remote site practice by new graduates, others require specific experience with the supervising physician prior to deployment to the remote site. Alaska, with the most geographically dispersed remote sites, is the most definitive about requirements for remote site practice.

> PAs in remote locations with less than 2 years of experience must first work 160 hours in direct patient care under immediate, direct supervision of collaborating or alternate collaborating physician. Periodic assessment for PAs with less than 2 years of experience must include at least one direct personal contact visit from supervising physician at least every 4 months for at least 4 hours.[1]

Kentucky requires newly graduated PAs must practice with on-site physician supervision for 18 months before they may practice in a location separate from the supervising physician. Colorado requires the onsite presence of a physician for the first 1000 hours of a new graduate's practice.[2]

Three states also require initial practice experience with the supervising physician even for experienced physician assistants. Kansas allows PAs to work in a separate location after 80 hours of work together. Mississippi requires the on-site presence of the supervising physician for the first 120 days. South Carolina requires six months clinical experience with the supervising physician before off-site supervision is authorized.[1]

States have a wide range of rules regarding the physician's presence in the remote site clinic. New Jersey and South Dakota are among the broadest with the "simple" requirement for "intermittent physical presence."

Missouri goes to the opposite extreme by requiring that the "Supervising physician must be present 66% of the time (per calendar quarter) PA is providing patient care." South Carolina is also at the "high end" of supervisory requirements by stating "the supervising physician must be physically present at least 20% of the time the PA is providing services."

Idaho, Montana, Nebraska, Tennessee, and North Carolina require monthly visits by supervising physicians. Pennsylvania, Oklahoma, Oregon, and Texas require an on-site visit every two weeks or every 10 business days. Monthly visits are a mandatory part of remote site supervision in Idaho, Montana Nebraska, Nevada, and Tennessee.

North Carolina is more specific by stipulating that the "PA must meet with supervising physician monthly for first 6 months of employment and every 6 months thereafter to discuss clinical problems and quality improvement measures."

With the growth and expansion of PA utilization, it's reasonable to expect that remote site practice by PAs and NPs will expand. Remote site is particularly relevant for small communities where closing hospitals make rural practice no longer feasible for physicians who need hospital practice to retain their procedural skills. Similarly, new patterns of care and the growing numbers of geriatric patients will expand what some states consider to be "remote site practice" in chronic care facilities, nursing homes, and hospice programs.

New technologies will also create new models of supervision. Already cell phones with photographic technology are being used to oversee HIV/AIDS treatment programs in Africa. Their application for clinician supervision—including the supervision of medical students and residents—has yet to be acknowledged. Similarly the supervision aspects of electronic medical records—including chart review and the monitoring of quality initiatives have yet to be built into the supervision methodologies for physician assistants and others.

REFERENCES

1. American Academy of Physician Assistants (AAPA) Web site. Summary of State Laws for Physician Assistants. Available at: http://www.aapa .org/advocacy-and-practice-resources/state-government-and-licensing/ state-laws-and-regulations/517-summary-of-state-laws-for-physician-assistants-abridged-version. Accessed January 2009.
2. AAPA Web site. Summary of State Laws for Physician Assistants Web site. Available at: http://www.aapa.org/advocacy-and-practice-resources/ state-government-and-licensing/state-laws-and-regulations/517-summary-of-state-laws-for-physician-assistants-abridged-version. Accessed January 2010.
3. AAPA Web site. Model State Legislation for Physician Assistants. Available at: http://www.aapa.org/advocacy-and-practice-resources/ state-government-and-licensing/state-laws-and-regulations/517-summary-of-state-laws-for-physician-assistants-abridged-version. Accessed January 2010.

Additional Resources

AAPA Code of Ethics
Source: http://www.aapa.org/advocacy-and-practice-resources/
practice-resources/ethics

AAPA Model Practice Act
Source: http://www.aapa.org/advocacy-and-practice-resources/
state-advocacy/490-model-state-legislation

Accreditation Standards for Physician Assistant Education©
(4th Edition)
Source: http://www.arc-pa.org/acc_standards

Code of Conduct for Certified and Certifying PAs
Source: http://www.nccpa.net/codeofconductlep.aspx

Competencies for the Physician Assistant Profession
Source: http://www.aapa.org/advocacy-and-practice-resources/
practice-resources/hospital-practice/557-pa-competency-measures

List and contact information of AAPA State Chapters
Source: http://www.aapa.org/partners/constituent-organizations/
chapters

List and contact information of PA postgraduate programs

Source: http://www.arc-pa.org/acc_programs/index.html

List and contact information of specialty PA organizations

Source: http://www.aapa.org/partners/constituent-organizations/specialty?view=places

List and contact Information of State Regulatory Boards

Source: http://www.fsmb.org/directory_smb.html

NCCPA Blueprint for PANCE & PANRE

Source: http://www.nccpa.net/examscontentblueprint.aspx

Sample Student Evaluation Instruments for Clinical Education

Arizona School of Health Sciences
Department of Physician Assistant Studies

MEDEX Northwest Division of
Physician Assistant Studies

Physician Assistant Training Program

Student Name _____   Preceptor _____

Rotation Site _____   Rotation # _____

Evaluate the following items with respect to the clinical rotation you just completed. Additional comments are encouraged, and are mandatory for any D or E rating.

Strongly Agree (A)   Agree (B)   Neutral (C)   Disagree (D)   Strongly Disagree (E)

Preceptor accepts/understands the PA concept.	A	B	C	D	E
Preceptor and/or staff provided orientation to the practice.	A	B	C	D	E
Preceptor provided timely feedback on task performance.	A	B	C	D	E
Preceptor held a formal evaluation session at mid-rotation.	A	B	C	D	E
Preceptor held a formal evaluation at the end of the rotation.	A	B	C	D	E
Preceptor helped me identify strengths and areas for improvement.	A	B	C	D	E
Preceptor assigned tasks appropriate to PA roles.	A	B	C	D	E
Preceptor directly observed me in patient encounters.	A	B	C	D	E
Preceptor provided opportunities to present patients.	A	B	C	D	E
Preceptor allowed me to discuss diagnostic studies and treatment options.	A	B	C	D	E
Preceptor was available for consultations when needed.	A	B	C	D	E
Preceptor allowed documentation of findings on charts.	A	B	C	D	E
Preceptor allowed me to perform complete history and physical exams.	A	B	C	D	E
Preceptor allowed me to perform diagnostic and therapeutic procedures.	A	B	C	D	E
Preceptor assigned topics for discussion or provided adequate informal teaching discussions.	A	B	C	D	E
This rotation allowed me to achieve the stated objectives.	A	B	C	D	E
My role as a student PA was accepted by Physicians and Residents.	A	B	C	D	E

My role as a student PA was accepted by nurses and technicians.	A	B	C	D	E
Overall, this rotation site provides a valuable learning experience.	A	B	C	D	E
Overall, the preceptor(s) for this rotation site is/are effective.	A	B	C	D	E
Are there any safety concerns with this site? (if yes, please explain below)	Yes		No		

What are the strengths of the site? _____
_____
_____

What are the weaknesses of the site? _____
_____
_____

Additional Comments: _____
_____
_____
_____
_____
_____
_____
_____
_____
_____
_____

Student Signature _____ Date _____

Mid-Term Physician Assistant Student Clinical Rotation Evaluation

Department of Physician Assistant
Studies
A.T. Still University
Arizona School of Health Sciences
5850 E. Still Circle
Mesa, AZ 85206
Phone: 480-219-6000
Fax: 480-219-6144

Student Name _____
Rotation 1 2 3 4 5 6 7 8
Clinical Site _____
Specialty _____
Primary Preceptor _____
Secondary Preceptor _____

Evaluate the student by circling the appropriate number in each category. Rate the student's level of proficiency based on his/her level of education, including both positive and negative comments. Please review the form with the student.

Clinical Performance	Excellent Satisfactory Poor
Demonstrates comprehension of material including understanding of anatomy and physiology, microbiology and pertinent pathophysiology of common problems; contributes as a positive member of the healthcare team; seeks consultation when indicated.	10 9 8 7 6 5 4 3 2 1 0 N/A Comments:

Interviewing and History Skills	Excellent Satisfactory Poor
Demonstrates appropriate communication skills and established rapport and respect while collecting a thorough history of acute and/or chronic problems from the CC, HPI, PMH, FH, Social HX, and ROS; collects history within the appropriate time frame while demonstrating sensitivity and compassion; identifies drug and other allergies.	10 9 8 7 6 5 4 3 2 1 0 N/A Comments:

Physical Exam Skills	Excellent	Satisfactory	Poor
Demonstrates a level of competency and proficiency with PE techniques; performs a systematic and organized PE within the appropriate time frame; recognizes normal from abnormal variants from the physical findings; demonstrates sensitivity and respect for the patient and the family.	10 9 8 7 6 5 4 3 2 1 0 N/A Comments:		

Diagnostics and Laboratory Studies	Excellent	Satisfactory	Poor
Demonstrates a level of competency and proficiency by identifying and recommending/ performing appropriate tests; understands and responds appropriately to acute/chronic and abnormal findings.	10 9 8 7 6 5 4 3 2 1 0 N/A Comments:		

Clinical Tasks and Technical Skills	Excellent	Satisfactory	Poor
Demonstrates increasing proficiency in performing clinical tasks and technical skills including venipuncture, IV injection, suturing, EKG. pap smear, hem occult, urine, hematological, LP and central line insertion; understands basic wound care management; utilizes clean and sterile technique properly.	10 9 8 7 6 5 4 3 2 1 0 N/A Comments:		

Assessment and Diagnosis	Excellent	Satisfactory	Poor
Accurately interprets data and formulates an appropriate differential diagnosis list and tentative diagnosis; appropriately interprets diagnostic studies to support or modify the tentative diagnosis; recognizes medical emergency situations and responds appropriately.	10 9 8 7 6 5 4 3 2 1 0 N/A Comments:		

Plan and Management	Excellent Satisfactory Poor
Shows independence and develops a comprehensive, safe, logical, and cost-effective plan based on the tentative and differential diagnosis list; demonstrates effective counseling skills; identifies appropriate therapeutic treatment plans based on knowledge of pharmacology for acute and chronic problems; develops a strategy for appropriate follow-up and/or referral.	10 9 8 7 6 5 4 3 2 1 0 N/A Comments:

Oral and Written Communication Skills	Excellent Satisfactory Poor
Demonstrates ability to effectively and completely communicate while counseling patients, presenting cases and documenting in the medical record; records and communicates data in an organized and concise manner; communicates pertinent clinical information when ordering diagnostic exams and referrals; effectively demonstrates ability to communicate through admission, comprehensive and problem focused H&Ps, SOAP and progress notes and discharge summaries.	10 9 8 7 6 5 4 3 2 1 0 N/A Comments:

Time Management and Assignments	Excellent Satisfactory Poor
Utilizes schedule to maximize learning opportunities; appropriately researches cases and completes reading and other assignments efficiently; reports for duty on time and is willing to adjust schedule to accommodate the preceptor; fulfills obligations, commitments and assignments in a timely manner.	10 9 8 7 6 5 4 3 2 1 0 N/A Comments:

Professionalism	Excellent Satisfactory Poor
Demonstrates a genuine interest in learning; wears appropriate identification (student, university, other); dresses appropriately while considering the clinical setting; nails, facial hair and long hair are clean and well-groomed; works cooperatively with staff and other healthcare professionals; always maintains patient confidentiality; maintains professional attitudes.	10 9 8 7 6 5 4 3 2 1 0 N/A Comments:

Judgment and Common Sense	Excellent Satisfactory Poor
Responds to clinical situations in a logical and responsible manner; establishes correct clinical and ethical priorities in patient care; demonstrates a high level of responsibility, ethical practice and sensitivity to a diverse patient population; adheres to all legal and regulatory requirements.	10 9 8 7 6 5 4 3 2 1 0 N/A Comments:

Summary Comments (strengths/weaknesses, suggested areas for improvement)	
Preceptor Signature _____	Total Hours (Primary Preceptor) _____
Date _____	Total Hours (Secondary Preceptor) _____
Student Signature _____	
Date _____	

Final Physician Assistant Student Clinical Rotation Evaluation

Department of Physician Assistant
Studies
A.T. Still University
Arizona School of Health Sciences
5850 E. Still Circle
Mesa, AZ 85206
Phone: 480-219-6000
Fax: 480-219-6144

Student Name _____
Rotation 1 2 3 4 5 6 7 8
Clinical Site _____
Specialty _____
Primary Preceptor _____
Secondary Preceptor _____

Evaluate the student by circling the appropriate number in each category. Rate the student's level of proficiency based on his/her level of education, including both positive and negative comments. Please review the form with the student.

Clinical Performance	Excellent Satisfactory Poor
Demonstrates comprehension of material including understanding of anatomy and physiology, microbiology and pertinent pathophysiology of common problems; contributes as a positive member of the healthcare team; seeks consultation when indicated.	10 9 8 7 6 5 4 3 2 1 0 N/A Comments:

Interviewing and History Skills	Excellent Satisfactory Poor
Demonstrates appropriate communication skills and established rapport and respect while collecting a thorough history of acute and/or chronic problems from the CC, HPI, PMH, FH, Social HX, and ROS; collects history within the appropriate time frame while demonstrating sensitivity and compassion; identifies drug and other allergies.	10 9 8 7 6 5 4 3 2 1 0 N/A Comments:

Physical Exam Skills	Excellent Satisfactory Poor
Demonstrates a level of competency and proficiency with PE techniques; performs a systematic and organized PE within the appropriate time frame; recognizes normal from abnormal variants from the physical findings; demonstrates sensitivity and respect for the patient and the family.	10 9 8 7 6 5 4 3 2 1 0 N/A Comments:

Diagnostics and Laboratory Studies	Excellent Satisfactory Poor
Demonstrates a level of competency and proficiency by identifying and recommending/ performing appropriate tests; understands and responds appropriately to acute/chronic and abnormal findings.	10 9 8 7 6 5 4 3 2 1 0 N/A Comments:

Clinical Tasks and Technical Skills	Excellent Satisfactory Poor
Demonstrates increasing proficiency in performing clinical tasks and technical skills including venipuncture, IV injection, suturing, EKG. pap smear, hem occult, urine, hematological, LP and central line insertion; understands basic wound care management; utilizes clean and sterile technique properly.	10 9 8 7 6 5 4 3 2 1 0 N/A Comments:

Assessment and Diagnosis	Excellent Satisfactory Poor
Accurately interprets data and formulates an appropriate differential diagnosis list and tentative diagnosis; appropriately interprets diagnostic studies to support or modify the tentative diagnosis; recognizes medical emergency situations and responds appropriately.	10 9 8 7 6 5 4 3 2 1 0 N/A Comments:

Plan and Management	Excellent Satisfactory Poor
Shows independence and develops a comprehensive, safe, logical, and cost-effective plan based on the tentative and differential diagnosis list; demonstrates effective counseling skills; identifies appropriate therapeutic treatment plans based on knowledge of pharmacology for acute and chronic problems; develops a strategy for appropriate follow-up and/or referral.	10 9 8 7 6 5 4 3 2 1 0 N/A Comments:

Oral and Written Communication Skills	Excellent Satisfactory Poor
Demonstrates ability to effectively and completely communicate while counseling patients, presenting cases and documenting in the medical record; records and communicates data in an organized and concise manner; communicates pertinent clinical information when ordering diagnostic exams and referrals; effectively demonstrates ability to communicate through admission, comprehensive and problem focused H&Ps, SOAP and progress notes and discharge summaries.	10 9 8 7 6 5 4 3 2 1 0 N/A Comments:

Time Management and Assignments	Excellent Satisfactory Poor
Utilizes schedule to maximize learning opportunities; appropriately researches cases and completes reading and other assignments efficiently; reports for duty on time and is willing to adjust schedule to accommodate the preceptor; fulfills obligations, commitments and assignments in a timely manner.	10 9 8 7 6 5 4 3 2 1 0 N/A Comments:

Professionalism	Excellent Satisfactory Poor
Demonstrates a genuine interest in learning; wears appropriate identification (student, university, other); dresses appropriately while considering the clinical setting; nails, facial hair and long hair are clean and well-groomed; works cooperatively with staff and other healthcare professionals; always maintains patient confidentiality; maintains professional attitudes.	10 9 8 7 6 5 4 3 2 1 0 N/A Comments:

Judgment and Common Sense	Excellent Satisfactory Poor
Responds to clinical situations in a logical and responsible manner; establishes correct clinical and ethical priorities in patient care; demonstrates a high level of responsibility, ethical practice and sensitivity to a diverse patient population; adheres to all legal and regulatory requirements.	10 9 8 7 6 5 4 3 2 1 0 N/A Comments:

Summary Comments (strengths/weaknesses, suggested areas for improvement)	
Preceptor Signature_____	Total Hours (Primary Preceptor) _____
Date _____	Total Hours (Secondary Preceptor) _____
Student Signature _____	
Date _____	

**To be completed by Student   Due: 1 week after each rotation

CLERKSHIP
SITE EVALUATION BY STUDENT

SAMPLE: You will normally complete this as an online form. Use this paper form only if you are experiencing technical difficulties.

Student: _____   Site/Clinic Name: _____

Preceptor: _____   Type of Rotation: _____

Date/from: _____ / _____   Length of time at site (weeks): _____

	Yes	No	Mixed Feelings
1. Were you expected and made to feel welcome?	____	____	____
2. Did you receive adequate supervision and teaching from your preceptor? Comments:	____	____	____
3. Were you allowed to write on charts?	____	____	____
4. Were you allowed to see patients alone?	____	____	____
5. Was your clerkship experience basically what you had wanted it to be? Please specify:	____	____	____
6. Were there any skills and/ or areas of knowledge in which you felt you should have been better prepared prior to clerkships? (Be specific) Skills: Knowledge:	____	____	____
7. Given your level of preparation going into clerkships, did the objectives seem reasonable? Please be specific if your answer is 'no' or 'mixed feelings.'	____	____	____
8. Were you able to achieve the objectives to your own satisfaction? Please be specific if your answer is 'no' or 'mixed feelings.'	____	____	____

9. **Required:** Please assess your strengths and weaknesses in this clerkship site at this stage in your clinical and professional development. (You have more strengths than weaknesses!)

STRENGTHS   WEAKNESSES

_____   _____

_____   _____

_____   _____

_____   _____

_____

_____

Rev. August 2009
University of Washington

**To be completed by Student   Due: Middle of Preceptorship
                                       (after eight weeks) Nov 12/June 17

PRECEPTORSHIP
FIRST EVALUATION OF PRECEPTOR

Student: _____   Preceptor: _____

Site: _____   Date: _____

	Always	Usually	Seldom
1. Does Your Preceptor:			
a. On 'patient presentation'			
1. Listen attentively			
2. Allow you to present completely	___	___	___
3. Encourage you to present completely	___	___	___
4. Critique your presentations	___	___	___
b. 'Take over' the care of the patients	___	___	___
How would you change this?			
c. Critique your charts			
What change would you like to see in this	___	___	___
procedure?			
d. Challenge your thinking by asking you to	___	___	___
explain your choice of diagnosis, treatment,			
alternatives			
What would you recommend?			
e. Accept diagnosis and treatment that vary from			
their established patterns			
1. When they are well defined by the student	___	___	___
2. Never vary from his or her tried and true	___	___	___
diagnosis and treatment			
f. Assign appropriate patients to student care	___	___	___
2. Describe Your Relationship To Your Preceptor:			
a. Authoritarian			
b. Collegial	___	___	___
c. Other: describe	___	___	___
	___	___	___

3. Would You Recommend Your Preceptor
To Other Students?
Explain:

4. What Changes Would You Recommend?
(*i.e.,* level of student responsibility, range of
patient age/problems, etc.)

5. Any Additional Comments You Wish To Make?

Rev. August 2010

**To be completed by Student   Due: End of Preceptorship
                                                              Jan 28/Aug 12

PRECEPTORSHIP
FIRST EVALUATION OF PRECEPTOR

Student: _____   Preceptor: _____

Site: _____   Date: _____

	Always	Usually	Seldom
1. Does Your Preceptor:			
a. On 'patient presentation'			
1. Listen attentively			
2. Allow you to present completely	___	___	___
3. Encourage you to present completely	___	___	___
4. Critique your presentations	___	___	___
b. 'Take over' the care of the patients	___	___	___
How would you change this?	___	___	___
c. Critique your charts			
What change would you like to see in this	___	___	___
procedure?			
d. Challenge your thinking by asking you to	___	___	___
explain your choice of diagnosis, treatment,			
alternatives			
What would you recommend?			
e. Accept diagnosis and treatment that vary			
from their established patterns	___	___	___
1. When they are well defined by the student	___	___	___
2. Never vary from his or her tried and true			
diagnosis and treatment	___	___	___
f. Assign appropriate patients to student care			
2. Describe Your Relationship To Your Preceptor:	___	___	___
a. Authoritarian	___	___	___
b. Collegial	___	___	___
c. Other: describe			

3. Would You Recommend Your Preceptor To
Other Students?
Explain:

4. What Changes Would You Recommend?
(*i.e.*, level of student responsibility, range of
patient age/problems, etc.)

5. Any Additional Comments You Wish To Make?

                                                              Rev. August 2010

**To be completed by student   Due: 1 week after visit

PRECEPTORSHIP
STUDENT EVALUATION OF SITE VISITOR

Student: _____   Date of Visit: _____
Site Visitor: _____   Preceptor: _____
                                            Site: _____

Summary of effect of site visit:

+3	+2	+1	0	-1	-2	-3
(positive effect)			(no effect)		(negative effect)	

Do you feel that your site visit demonstrated a clear picture of your preceptorship situation?
Please be specific. _____
_____
_____
_____

Was your site visitor effective in resolving issues with your preceptor?
Please discuss specifics. _____
_____
_____
_____

Was your site visitor effective in resolving issues with the office staff?
_____
_____
_____

Did your site visitor provide you with adequate support at the site visit?
Please discuss specifics. _____
_____
_____
_____

Any other comments? (Use back of page if necessary.)
_____
_____
_____

What thoughts or considerations were expressed by your preceptor concerning the visit of the site visitor?

_____

_____

_____

_____

Were you in agreement with your on-site evaluation and recommendations? If not, what additional comments and/or suggestions would you make?

_____

_____

_____

_____

Rev. August 2009   University of Washington

Index

Note: Figures are indicated with an italicized page-locator; tables are noted with a *t*.